HEALTH CARE:
INNOVATION, IMPACT AND CHALLENGE

HEALTH CARE:

INNOVATION, IMPACT AND CHALLENGE

Edited by

S. Mathwin Davis

School of Policy Studies/School of Public Administration
Queen's University

Canadian Cataloguing in Publication Data

Main entry under title:

Health care : innovation, impact and challenge

Papers presented at a conference held at Queen's University in June 1992.
ISBN 0-88911-639-3

1. Medical care - Canada - Congresses. 2. Public health - Canada -
Congresses. 3. Medical care, Cost of - Canada - Congresses. 4. Public
health - Canada - Finance - Congresses. I. Davis, Sturton Mathwin,
1919-   . II. Queen's University (Kingston, Ont.). School of Public
Administration. III. Queen's University (Kingston, Ont.). School of
Policy Studies.

RA449.H4 1992   362.1'09714   C92-095765-X

Cover Photo   Alasdair Roberts
                School of Public Administration, Queen's University

For our daughters
Diane Felicity and Deborah Lynn

Contents

CHALLENGE

INITIATIVES

Preface

Some of our readers may have been present at the last conference of this nature given at Queen's in 1989. At that time, the title "Healthy Populace, Healthy Policy — Medicare Toward the Year 2000" seemed to imply that — given the right decisions, i.e., "The best policies" — Medicare could move steadily ahead until the turn of the century. Back in 1989 we were perhaps not as prescient as we might have been. It was, so to speak, as if

> All heedless of the danger
> The little lambkins play
> They do not hear the warning
> And live but for today.

Clearly, in 1992, the situation is somewhat different. It is often reported that health care is in a crisis — but it is believed that this is an understatement. Hopefully we could emerge from a crisis and go on to greater things. In our case, however, we do not face an ephemeral perturbation but, rather, the need to address and adapt to an ongoing, changed, and much more financially responsible situation. Thus, while our *policies* may be admirable and well intentioned, it is their successful and prudently exercised implementation that must be our current objective.

Accordingly, the title of our present conference "Health Care — Innovation, Impact and Challenge" does, we hope, reflect a reasonably enlightened awareness of our present concerns. The challenges surround us, their rising costs assail us on all sides and we must try — not infrequently with a certain desperation — to develop innovative concepts and actions that will enable us to continue to provide, at the minimum, an adequate level of health care. It is these sentiments, therefore, that have motivated the design of the conference, an approach that we hope you will find appropriate.

The general pattern of the deliberations has been comprehensively outlined in Duncan Sinclair's introduction. And the papers themselves are generally as they were presented, with appropriate editing from the audio-visual record. As an innovation at this conference, we arranged for a series of demonstration booths that elicited an excellent response from those who were concerned to describe their own "innovations." Several of these made short presentations, which have been included in this report.

It is appropriate, at the outset, to record the many areas of support that have made the conference possible. Particularly we are indebted to the Health Policy Research & Evaluation Unit of Community Health and Epidemiology at Queen's as well as to the Teaching Health Unit for significant financial contributions, so that we could be cost efficient but not parsimonious. Since both these contributions emanate from the Ministry of Health we must also gratefully acknowledge their support.

Clearly the success of the conference — and several individuals made it a point to say that it *was* a success — is due in large measure to the high quality of the papers presented and we are most happy to acknowledge this. No less do we appreciate the unseen, but very significant contributions from staff members of the School of Policy Studies/School of Public Administration — Margaret Innes, Marilyn Redmond, Jane Hodgins, Lynn Freeman, Mary Kennedy and Valerie Jarus.

And, over more than twelve months, a Working Group laboured over a wealth of high policy and administrative detail.

Most particularly, however, I would like to express the warmest personal appreciation for the ongoing administrative and editorial endeavours of Marilyn Banting. Without her skilled assistance neither the conference nor this book would have been accomplished. Indeed, her only failing is that she would not allow her name to be credited as co-editor. This, however, may be a good thing since any errors are quite clearly mine and not hers.

As Canadians, we have a health-care system that is admirable — and the envy of many in North America. If, as is appearing to be the case, we have somewhat over-reached ourselves then it is appropriate that we recall Browning's sentient observation

> ... Man's reach should exceed his grasp,
> Or what's a Heaven for?

Noting prudently, but perhaps less poetically, that it would be more appropriate to observe "People's reach etc. etc. — it is pertinent to echo his question. Our hope is that the deliberations of this conference — while perhaps not providing a Heavenly benediction — will, in some measure have helped to show us the way.

S. Mathwin Davis
Conference Chairman

Conference Working Group

Dr. S. Mathwin Davis
Conference Chairman
School of Public Administration
Queen's University

Mr. John Dorland
Health Policy Research &
Evaluation Unit
Queen's University

Mr. Mark Edmonds
Director of Diagnostic &
Patient Services
Hotel Dieu Hospital
Kingston, Ontario

Dr. David Mowat
Medical Officer of Health
Kingston, Frontenac and Lennox
& Addington Health Unit

Dr. David Bray
Health Policy Research &
Evaluation Unit
Queen's University

Ms Ena Howse
School of Nursing
Queen's University

Mr. Ahsan Sadiq
Senior Consultant
Claims Payment Operations
Ministry of Health

Introduction

Duncan G. Sinclair

It is a daunting challenge to be asked to introduce the theme of a conference on health care with such an all encompassing title as "Innovation, Impact and Challenge." In fact, there is very little that would not be included were I to take my assignment literally.

There are some parallels with the Premier of Ontario's Council on Health, Well-Being and Social Justice. It is hard to conceive of any aspect of human endeavour that does not fall within the combined mandate of both the Premier's Council and the Council on Economic Renewal.

The papers in this volume focus on the most significant of the many challenges facing health care and describe the impact of innovations we must make to continue to provide the public with steadily improving access to health care that will increase, in ways we can afford, their health and well-being. I need say little about the impact of health care. All of us know a good deal about the fact that we Canadians spend more money per capita on our health-care system than any other country in the world, apart from the United States, and the most of any country with a publicly-financed system. In aggregate, spending on health care eats up something close to a third of the budget of provinces like Ontario and the proportion continues to grow, slowed in its rate of increase only recently by dint of application of some very hard-nosed policies commonly referred to as caps, cutbacks, and clawbacks — all words signifying the end of further increases in the share of the public purse spent on health care. Basically, this decision has been taken because it is apparent that the impact of health-care spending on other necessary social investments — education, roads, bridges, and other infrastructures, technology, communication, social assistance, child care, pay and employment equity, new business development, etc., the list is very long — is negative and too great!

The taxpayer, living as he or she does right next to the United States, has concluded that enough is enough and will not tolerate any decrease in his or her present standard of living to support happily more spending on Canada's famed social safety net. So increasing the total pie is not a viable option for governments to maintain the growth in spending on health care to which we who use the system have been accustomed for many years.

So innovation is the order of the day. We are going to have to learn how to do things differently, how to be more efficient — that is, get more effective health care delivered to the people who need it for the dollars we have available. I am reminded of Lord Rutherford's famous comment when the budget to support his laboratory's research on splitting the atom ran out. "Gentlemen," (and they were all gentlemen then), "we have no money. We'll have to think!"

One of the things we have been thinking about in the last few years is how much societal benefit are we getting for all the money we spend on the health-care system. As the accountants say, we have been doing a sort of value-for-money audit. As most of us know well, the results have not been such as to make us all swell with pride or the Canadian taxpayer believe that he or she has access to the best health-care system in the world. It is true that all we have available to us are very crude indicators such as: length of life, infant mortality, survival to specific ages, and the like. But it remains, according to these crude indicators, that the health status of Canadians is, on average, nothing like second in the world, a rank that would match our spending on health care. We have respectable statistics but certainly nothing to crow about in terms of a value-for-money audit. In fact, the only consolation to us is that the Americans, who spend more, apparently get even less value. Frankly, that is neither a high standard nor a comparison to console us!

So we need some innovative thinking! We will start with three presentations of contemporary innovations.

Dr. John Marshall, my friend and colleague from Queen's Academic Medical Centre, will speak on the application of Kaizen, Total Quality Management, Continuous Quality Improvement — there are many words and phrases to describe this new approach to finding better ways of doing things — to the individuals and institutions that make up the health-care system.

John will be followed by Drs. Woodward and Curry who will describe a new approach to capturing information about encounters between patients and the health-care system — the health encounter card. It is rather sobering to think as innovative the determination to collect reliable information about the services patients demand and get from the system, the same one that costs us a third of provincial revenues and such a high proportion of our GNP. But the plain facts are that this hugely expensive and cherished system does not now have the capacity to yield the information to allow us to judge the extent to which we are getting value for our expenditures. I can assure you that heads would roll in a comparable private-sector business with costs even a fraction of the $17 billions that health care costs in Ontario alone! So it is really quite innovative to be talking about ways of keeping track of what we are buying with our health-care dollars.

The third paper, by Dr. Pineault of the Université de Montréal, describes policy changes in Quebec designed to increase the efficiency of the system; make it more effective, especially in terms of improving access to the health-care system in under-serviced parts of the province; and to make the whole system more responsive to the perceived needs of its consumers — patients and the populations and communities from which they come. Our colleagues in Quebec have a long record of leading us all in innovative ways of managing the health-care system from a public policy perspective. *La belle province* recognized before the rest of us that health care is a public good and the health-care system, in effect, a regulated public utility. Innovative management in a public utility should not be an oxymoron. We look forward to Dr. Pineault's description of why it makes sense.

I remind you again of the title of this conference, "Health Care — Innovation, Impact and Challenge." There are many challenges one can think of, but one that is very important must surely be the reforming of health-care financing in the United States. To borrow a quotation from the Desert Storm exercise, Dr. Woolhander's topic is in the "mother-of-all-challenges" category. Our challenge here in Canada of getting more efficiency and effectiveness out of our health-care system and keeping it within the limits of what we can afford does not really measure up to the challenge of trying to develop a system so that all members of the richest nation on earth have access to at least a basic level of health-care services. A few weeks ago, Mark Gibson, Executive Assistant to the President of the Senate in the State of Oregon, visited Queen's and spoke to us about the so-called Oregon experiment in making medicaid and medicare benefits universally available within the state. When he was asked by a member of the audience if he was concerned about the consequences of having a two-tiered system, he replied that he regarded getting to a two-tiered system as a tremendous accomplishment for the people of Oregon. He explained that now there are multiple tiers with the bottom being a substantial number of the most needy, and at risk of having no access at all to health services.

So that is innovation. What about impact?

The next section features impact. Speaking from the perspective of the consumer, as she has done so credibly and successfully for so many years, will be Joan Watson. Presenting the perspective of the Ministry of Health, the people on the firing line, facing consumers and taxpayers on one side and providers of health care on the other, Michael Decter, Deputy Minister of Health for Ontario. Both will speak to health-care issues as they are developing in Ontario but I am sure the issues will be directly applicable to all other provinces and to the nation as a whole.

Michael Decter's challenge — his job — is said to be the most difficult in the province. His ministry spends more money than any other in the provincial government and, of course, it is to Health that his colleagues and everyone else looks when money is tight and they want to save some for other purposes. Yet it is also to Health that both providers and consumers look when anything goes wrong and they get worried about their access to health-care services. Some months ago the province of Ontario decided no longer to insure depilation, hair removal. One had the mental image of Michael Decter and Bob MacMillan, Director of OHIP, being chased through the halls of the Hepburn Block by a mob of angry, hirsute people out onto Grosvenor Street, right into the arms of a crowd of irate dermatologists. He can certainly talk to us about impact.

But Joan Watson's is the greater challenge. There are approaching 30 million consumers in Canada and she has to speak for us all. To be fair, she will only speak to current developments in Ontario from the perspective of the 9 million or so consumers who live in this province; but still, speaking on behalf of 9 million people is no joke, especially when you know they do not all hold the same views.

And that is one of the greatest challenges facing the health-care system. The system is here, after all, to serve the people who need it and who pay for it. Those people have quite remarkably different points of view and the health-care system when they approach it as a patient, or the parent or child of a patient, or as a patient's friend and advocate. They are very knowledgeable, on the whole, about modern technology and services. They are well aware that Canada is said to have one of, it not *the* best health-care system in the world and they want, quite understandably, full access to the full spectrum of what they think it can and should accomplish. They are not terribly patient with discussions about Resource Intensity Weights, Long-Term Care Reform, and the Evans, Spassoff and Podborsky Reports when they think Johnny needs to go through the MRI after falling out of the swing on his head or Grannie isn't admitted after her dizzy spell. The same consumer, of course, is also a member of the alliance against tax increases and of the car pool to the Salmon Run Mall in upstate New York each weekend to buy the groceries.

Joan Watson's challenge is considerable!

Finally, I will conclude with some words about academic medicine, nursing, rehabilitation, and all the other health professional faculties and schools of the universities, colleges, and teaching hospitals of Canada.

When it comes to innovation, on one side of our house we have a great deal to be proud of. I speak, of course, about biomedical science. Since those early days of this century when Abraham Flexner and the American Medical Association initiated the reforms that put medicine and the other health professions on the road to their present scientific foundation, we in Canada have accomplished much. Banting and Best's discovery of insulin remains, of course, our most prominent contribution to knowledge of how to apply scientific understanding to prevent and treat disease; but there have been many other contributions by scientists working in the health professional faculties, schools and hospitals of Canada. They make it possible for us to say we have paid our way in advancing human understanding of how human beings function in health, how diseases alter those functions, and how to react and heal the sick. Canada's physicians, nurses, rehabilitationists, dentists, pharmacists — the whole spectrum of those who make the health-care system function — are well educated and superbly trained, able to compare favourably with their counterparts anywhere in the world. We have much of which to be very proud!

Innovative as we have been in biomedical research and in educating our successors, we have not been very good at developing innovations leading to cost-containment or savings, in making available health-care services of increasing complexity and sophistication within the limits of what our society can afford to pay on behalf of those Canadians who need them. To be fair, until very recently nobody seemed to care very much about research in the cost-effectiveness of health care, including the governments that insured the system. Certainly then, as now, the academic health professional faculties and schools have had to struggle mightily to secure funds, first to expand the number of people with expertise in this kind of work, second to support their work, and third, to develop the kind of data systems to capture raw material about the nature of encounters between individual patients and their physicians, nurses, rehabilitationists, dentists, pharmacists, hospitals, community clinics, and so on. Again, I return to the theme that the private sector business that had as little information about its customers as the publicly-funded health-care system would not stay in business very long!

But it remains that the academic health professions' record of innovativeness in making the health-care system optimally cost-effective, has been much less than our society needs from us. Our universities and related educational institutions are, after all, set up by society to be proactive, to conduct research and scholarly work at the leading edge, to *lead* society, not react to the blunt instruments of government's budgets, constraints, cutbacks to achieve societal change — the very instruments to which we are now reacting with such pain and suffering. It is our responsibility to foresee and lead social change, not react to it — and in this our record is not one of which I, for one, am very proud.

But neither is it one of which I am embarrassed. We are on the move and have shifted into the highest gear we have been able to run in, given the constraints within which the academic and research community of Canada has had to live for many years. Ontario's universities, by the way, are funded least well of those in all Canada's provinces and Canadian universities as a whole are funded at a fraction of research universities in the United States. So when I say that we have not done and are not doing what Canadian society should expect of the academic health professions in the development of new, innovative, imaginative approaches to health-care delivery that will enhance the quality of the system and yet be within our ability to pay, my statement should be put in the context of the old adage, "you get what you pay for." We have produced in spades value for money in biomedical research. We have probably also done so in health services research but it remains that much, much more is needed if we are to meet the challenges of the Canadian health-care system as we close out the twentieth and enter the twenty-first century.

This volume addresses the important issues of today. It acts as a stepping stone to our meeting the challenges of health care in Canada.

NATIONAL POLICIES

1

Review of Provincial Systems

Raisa Deber, Ross Baker and Sharmila Mhatre

Medicare is, yet again, in crisis. The good news is that there does seem to be a national consensus on something — the diagnosis seems relatively constant from province to province. The bad news is that the consensus appears to be that Medicare is in bad shape; certainly the rhetoric, if not necessarily the system, is fevered.

This paper is intended to give a general overview of the current Canadian scene, noting how the provinces are attempting to meet the current crisis. The material will not be comprehensive, but should serve as a useful backdrop for the other papers.

Now, the first step of a diagnostician is to put the right fancy label on. And we would like to suggest that there has been a bit of misdiagnosis. Analysts are fond of suggesting that the problem is costs — rising at above the rate of inflation — and that we will have to scale back to a system we can afford. We hear lots of rhetoric about the need to make tragic choices, adopt Oregon-style models, and in general restrict government-financed services to what we can afford, perhaps with insurance companies and U.S. providers poised to pick up the slack.

We would like to suggest that this is a woefully premature prescription which, if adopted, is likely to kill the patient. Instead, we propose that the real problem confronting Canada's health-care system is appropriateness — both in what is delivered, and in how it is delivered. Appropriateness is a tough problem to deal with, not least because, as Bob Evans has pointed out, health costs are also health incomes.[1] If we get serious about ensuring that only appropriate care is delivered, there is likely to be significant loss of jobs, prestige to communities, professional income, and convenience to the public.

In the interim, it is well known that the easiest way to contain costs is to shift them. Table 1:1 presents our conceptualization — based in part on a paper by Paul Starr — of health-care systems.[2]

Table 1:1. *Classification of Health Care Systems*

FINANCING DELIVERY	Public	Private
Public	U.K.	–
Private	Canada	U.S.

Source: Authors' compilation.

There are two key elements here: first, the distinction between public and private; and second, between financing health care and the method of delivering health care.

Temporarily ignoring the fact that any actual system is a mixture of elements and will deviate from these "ideal types," we can classify the old National Health Services (NHS) system in the United Kingdom as public financing and public delivery, the neo-classical economists' version of the U.S. system (which, of course, is not what they really have) as private financing and private delivery, and the Canadian compromise as public financing and private delivery. As an aside, it is interesting to note the one blank cell in this matrix — no system of which we are aware has opted for private financing of a publicly delivered system.

However, if one tries to use this simple table, one finds that it does not provide enough detail to capture the sorts of changes and reforms that are happening in many health-care systems.

Deber, with Orvill Adams and Lynn Curry, has further developed this schema to distinguish levels of public and private, which apply to both the financing and delivery dimensions.[3] We break down *public* into four levels:

- the nation (e.g., the federal Canadian government)
- the state or province

- the region, and

- the locality.

Private can also be split into four levels:

- a series of charitable, non-profit "mediating institutions" (a category that would include most Canadian hospitals and social agencies)

- a small business/entrepreneurial sector (which in Canada would include most physicians)

- a corporate for-profit sector (which is most important in Canada for drugs and devices, but plays a major role in U.S. health care), and

- the family/personal sector, which is truly private in both senses of the word.

Some of the interesting policy developments occurring in recent years can be viewed as shifts *within* rather than between the public and private sectors. For example, the issue of which level of government should be responsible for what activities is important in many countries, and regional experiments abound. Within Canada, active issues include the balance among national, provincial, and regional responsibilities for financing of health-care services. Where "privatization" occurs, it is usually to the non-profit "mediating institutions," which perform quasi-governmental functions and operate under powerful government guidelines (e.g., the sickness funds of Western Europe; and the U.K. experiments with setting up hospital trusts). With the exception of the United States, there is little interest in transferring activities from the public to the for-profit sectors. However, there is also evidence of shifting among the private sector. One example is the proposed reforms of long-term care, which may imply that we are shifting responsibilities for delivery of care from the charitable mediating institutions back to the family.

These changes are operating within a fiscal context. Internationally, most industrialized countries are eager to curb the proportion of national wealth that is spent to purchase health-care services. In Canada, an additional dimension is the transition in financing from the national to the provincial governments, which began with the passage of Established Programs Financing (EPF) in 1977, and has accelerated in recent years. This distinction becomes particularly important in Canada, where health care is constitutionally the responsibility of the province, although the national government had taken responsibility for financing it, and for setting national standards.[4] As we rethink our federal system, we have increasingly had to ask "what happens to Medicare?" or, to put it another way: "If the Canadian ship of state sinks, do we have to jettison Medicare?"

A background paper for the HEAL lobby[5] summarizes some of the issues and categorizes roles the federal government might adopt.

Table 1:2.   *Potential Federal Roles in Health Care*

---

1.   ROLES LIKELY TO BE ASSUMED BY FEDERAL GOVERNMENT RE-
      GARDLESS OF CONSTITUTIONAL MODEL SELECTED

   A.   *Safety and Monitoring*
   B.   *Inter-provincial and international*

2.   ROLES LIKELY TO BE ASSUMED BY FEDERAL GOVERNMENT UNDER
      ALL BUT HIGHLY DEVOLVED CONSTITUTIONAL MODELS

   A.   *Research*
   B.   *Training*
   C.   *Financing*

3.   ROLES LIKELY TO BE ASSUMED BY FEDERAL GOVERNMENT IF A
      SUBSTANTIAL FEDERAL ROLE RETAINED; OTHERWISE MAY BE AS-
      SUMED BY OTHER NATIONAL BODIES

   A.   *Coordination (could be strong or weak)*
   B.   *Policy guidance*
   C.   *Information clearing house*
   D.   *Setting national standards*

4.   ROLES LIKELY TO BE ABANDONED BY FEDERAL GOVERNMENT,
      REGARDLESS OF CONSTITUTIONAL MODEL ADOPTED

   A.   *Service delivery*

Source: Authors' compilation.

If, then, the federal government is likely to shed a number of its traditional roles — and enforcing national standards may indeed be one of them — what happens?

One obvious distinction is that there are things that should be done at a national level (although they are not necessarily being done), but these activities may not have to be *federal* responsibilities. A good deal of the coordination is currently being done within such federal-provincial mechanisms as the Conference of Deputy Ministers of Health and its subcommittee structure; this has mixed effectiveness. If the federal government chooses to abandon certain roles, we are going to need new structures, and/or to strengthen existing ones. Examples of these already exist — the Canadian Coordinating Office on Health Technology Assessment (CCOTA), and the MIS Group. Many of the most effective ones are essentially ad hoc. In that connection, it is interesting to note that despite the absence of formal coordinating mechanisms, there was a high degree of consensus on the policy directions that emerged from the recent slew of provincial commissions; key themes have been summarized in recent papers by Doug Angus, and by Mhatre and Deber.[6] One can speculate that these may be related to the ease of informal communications — particularly, the existence of telephones, fax machines, and Bob Evans.

To summarize, there are some common problems in Canada's health-care system. Costs keep rising at a higher rate than inflation, and control efforts to date resemble squeezing a balloon — curbs in one place appear to lead to increases in others. There are also a number of common reactions that have occurred in the various provinces.

We have divided up the changes we see happening into six broad categories.

The first is *changes in financing*, that is, how can the provinces get more money to pay for Medicare? At this moment, the federal government does not look like a very promising source. Indeed, if one extrapolates current trends, the cash portion of EPF will vanish.[7] There is still a substantial degree of federal transfer payments, but much of this is not in the form of cash, and hence is not in a form that gives Ottawa much leverage over provincial policies.

Moving back to our classification of health systems, we can question whether these financing methods are tied to service delivery. One group of financing methods are tied: it includes not only the obvious direct charges (e.g., extra-billing), but also other proposed user fees (e.g., Quebec's threat to charge $5 to patients making "unnecessary" visits to emergency rooms). These sorts of charges for insured services are clearly violations of the *Canada Health Act* (CHA), and most provinces have indicated they reject them, at least for the present. (Although both Saskatchewan and Quebec have publicly mused about the possibility. Unfortunately, direct charges seem to be what Bob Evans calls zombies — ideas that should be dead, but keep walking around and doing damage.)[8] We would also argue that the proposals to make the value of medical care a taxable benefit are equivalent to direct charges, albeit ones more easily geared to income. Administratively, they are not levied at the point of service, which would appear to make them even less likely to affect utilization and more likely to constitute a pure tax on illness. Accordingly, although they might not legally be deemed violations of the principles of Medicare and of the *Canada Health Act,* morally, they clearly appear to be.

A broader issue is whether the federal government chooses to enforce the CHA. At present, they do not seem that anxious to. The reasons for this may stem from a reluctance to penalize provinces whose support is needed on other issues, or a lack of confidence that the sanctions available will effect any meaningful change.

There are also a number of ways provinces can increase revenues that have nothing to do with service receipt, but which governments like to link to health for optical reasons — that is, they are likely to get less public opposition to what is really just a tax increase. One example is Ontario's Employer's Health Tax, which, despite its name, is just a payroll tax whose only relationship to Medicare is its name. Similarly, premiums are just another tax as long as there is no connection between payment of premiums and eligibility to receive services.

We should note that although some think of these charges only as revenue sources, others talk of them as steering mechanisms which could be used to discourage certain types of activities. Quebec's $5 emergency room fee, for example, was described as a way of getting people to use more appropriate forms of care, such as CLSCs. However, this sort of fee is a pretty indirect way to do it, particularly because user fees are well known to discourage both appropriate and inappropriate care. They are also expensive to collect, particularly if the collector has to do an appropriateness review first! We would therefore argue that their only advantage is that they fit the ideology of private medicine — i.e., they cater to the assumption that people will abuse "free services." Since visiting the doctor is not my idea of fun, and since we argue that early detection of some things gives far better results, it is not clear why advocates of direct charges remain so convinced that having patients make these sorts of calculations is a useful exercise; they seem unlikely to have much impact unless they are so poor that the money really is a deterrent, in which case most proponents of user fees plan to waive them anyhow.

Government is not only trying to collect more, they are also trying to spend less. Between one-quarter and one-third of provincial budgets are now going for health, and all provinces seem to agree that that is enough. The second category of change is *changes in coverage.* Every province is looking at what they insure, and most are looking at their fee schedules. Comprehensiveness is defined in terms of medical necessity in the CHA, which leaves considerable room for debate as to what services must be included. At present, most provinces are making coverage decisions by looking at what the other provinces cover. So far, these appear to be based less on a coherent view of what is "medically required" or "necessary" and more on a sense of staying relatively similar to the other provinces. We could refer to this phenomenon as "keeping down with the Joneses." The targets for de-insurance to date appear to be such activities as cosmetic surgery, mental health, and things dealing with reproductive care, plus anything not required under the terms of the *Canada Health Act* (e.g., things other than doctors and hospitals). Ontario, for example, de-insured some cosmetic surgery, electrolysis for facial hair, and has taken aim at psychotherapy, IVF, labs, chiropractic, and the drug benefit plan. Alberta proposed to de-insure a wide variety of services, including many related to reproductive care (sterilization, etc.), although it has backed off on at least some. It also raised co-payments for the elderly for assistive devices and drugs.

The provinces are also clamping down on out-of-province coverage. Portability imposes some requirements for coverage within Canada (although Quebec is probably in violation of this), but less requirements for out-of-country coverage. Ontario, for example, went from being very generous to "snowbirds" to very generous to insurers; Ontario residents leaving the country had better take out private insurance or they could be in terrible financial trouble if they have a medical emergency. We have hypothesized that there may actually be a master plan here — although one that has gotten insufficient media attention — to use this threat as a secret weapon against cross-border shopping.

De-insurance so far has been pretty minimal. However, at its extreme, some people are now looking at the model proposed by Oregon, which in effect specifies a short list of "necessary" services and says that the poor — the only ones who would be affected by this model — will be on their own for everything else.[9] We predict that the concept of what care is "necessary" will get more attention, and Eleanor Ross and Raisa Deber are currently examining this issue.

A third development is *changes in delivery.* On one level, this encompasses simple attempts to downsize. A large number of beds have been removed from the system in Ontario — Toronto alone had taken over 2,800 beds out of service by August 1990.[10] New Brunswick has suggested that it will cut 400 beds in the next two years — about 10 percent of its total complement. Newfoundland has also closed hospital beds. Indeed, the phenomenon is nationwide.

But provinces are not just cutting; a more interesting development is trying to use downsizing to catalyze long-overdue changes in how services are organized. There has been considerable reexamination of the old model of the independent hospital and the independent fee-for-service physician, each deciding what their patients "needed" and leaving government to pick up the bill.

There are two major themes in this reexamination. The first is the move from institutions to the community, a shift which technological changes are making much easier. For example, it is now possible to do things on an outpatient or ambulatory basis that used to need hospitalization. British Columbia, for example, gave major increases to community services, mental health, and public health in its most recent budget while trying to curb hospital budgets. Every province is at least paying lip service to this concept.

The second theme is to eliminate waste and duplication. Provinces increasingly are recognizing that they may improve quality and cut costs through regionalization to eliminate duplication and set up centres of excellence. Although all the provincial reports and commissions talked about regional approaches, certain provinces are well ahead of the others on this. For example, British Columbia has done a lot on regionalization, as has Quebec. One of the influential national models is the Victoria Health Project, which we understand has now emerged from pilot project status to be a permanent planning and coordinating body. Although it is a strategy with considerable potential, it must also be recognized that appropriate referral/catchment areas will vary by service, and may not necessarily coincide with regional boundaries. To some extent, regionalization can be counterproductive if it forces the duplication of tertiary facilities within each region and discourages broader-based centres of excellence. A regional strategy also requires that one curb the power of individual institutions, and they can be *very* powerful. However, concrete action is occurring. New Brunswick abolished all 51 hospital boards and set up a series of eight regional boards. During the interim phase, the minister of health acted as hospital czar. Despite the furor, the government took over effective ownership of hospitals. Among the issues arising in such changes is the implication for the continuing mission of Catholic health care.

Saskatchewan also abolished individual boards and set up a provincially-appointed governance structure for Regina and Saskatoon. These new Health Boards are now responsible for governance of hospitals, major long-term care facilities, and home-care programs; the previous boards of these facilities have been dissolved. CEOs now have to report to the board president, who is appointed by the government. The new structure abolished VPs within the individual institutions for such things as finance, human resources, support services, medicine, nursing, continuing care, or community services; these have become corporate functions. As of this writing, the futures of people now holding those jobs in the individual institutions are therefore in doubt. To the extent that no mechanisms will be put in place to ensure accountability to the public — and this is by no means clear — Saskatchewan could be seen as moving towards the U.K. model of public financing and public delivery, a decided break with Canadian practice.

How well this will work remains very unclear, particularly since it was imposed on institutions rather than arising from their own efforts. There is currently a great deal of uncertainty, especially with CEOs used to charting their own missions. In addition, the informational requirements for the "super board" are clearly higher than they would be for the individual institutions, and new mechanisms may have to be devised to ensure that this information is available. A still unanswered question is whether these sorts of models will be given one communal budget with which to finance the full continuum of regional services. An advantage of this approach is that it may make labour adjustments easier; for example, a single budget may make it easier to cut facilities and move people into the community. A disadvantage is that pay scales are very different in these sectors; bringing all community-based salaries up to institutional levels is likely to be very expensive. It is not clear how the provinces plan to cope with these labour market issues involved in the transition.

To date, Ontario is considerably behind the rest of the country in eliminating this sort of duplication, probably because it was rich enough to avoid having to bite that particular bullet. However, even Ontario is now musing a bit about these sorts of regional solutions. One example is the Orser Report on Southwestern Ontario[11] which proposed a regional level of governance and a regional funding envelope, but also proposed adding a lot more capital money to sweeten the pot, which may be one reason why it seems stalled at present. The model proposed in Orser is also quite complex; it highlights the difficulty of balancing "community needs," the interests of key power blocks, and the interests of the region as a whole.

Voluntary efforts are also occurring. There is interesting progress by a group of community hospitals in the Toronto district of Scarborough, who have agreed in principle to a common board structure (based on the approval of each facility's board) and are now considering voluntary rationalization of their programs. This effort was sparked by the medical staffs, who want to consolidate services without losing their privileges, and feel that by reducing administrative duplication they might have more money left for clinical services. This is a very encouraging development, particularly if you think the purpose of health care is to take care of patients. Another group of hospitals in the west end of Toronto is also talking, and even the downtown teaching hospitals have formed a new coordinating structure.

On the other hand, the Ontario government is reopening the *Public Hospitals Act*.[12] Although this process is very much in flux, the current statement of guiding principles seems to have a difficult time reconciling the desire to respect the mission and tradition of individual institutions with any regional framework. One of the proposals — that each institution develop a "social contract" with its community — would make regional solutions even more difficult by entrenching the mission statements (and employment patterns) of each institution. It is not clear what is going to happen.

There are also fascinating developments concerning regionalization in Quebec, which are discussed by Dr. Pineault in this volume.

Other attempts being used in some provinces to change the way services are delivered include the series of provincial royal commissions and inquiries mentioned earlier, and a series of new corporatist advisory mechanisms (e.g., Premier's Councils) which can dilute the power of doctors and hospitals. Whether these are influential will depend on political factors. For example, Ontario's Premier's Council had its mission changed when the NDP government took power. It has taken on a representative/participatory rather than corporatist structure. Although there may be advantages to this change, it should be recognized that, on balance, the current council has less powerful members and a focus that is less interested in health care than in broader determinants of well-being; accordingly, it is less likely to be a major player in health policy development. Nova Scotia is also using a Premier's Council related to the older Ontario model; its influence remains to be seen. British Columbia has set up an elaborate secretariat within government to implement the recommendations of its Royal Commission on Health Care and Costs, and sounds like it is very serious about system reform.

The fourth trend is *changes in the way one deals with providers,* particularly physicians. Doctor bashing is in, in part because doctors are the gatekeepers to an expensive system. There appear to be three widely-held articles of faith among provincial governments. The first is that there are too many doctors. The Barer-Stoddart Report got a lot of play. The second is that these doctors are badly distributed. There is considerable attention to how to get a better distribution, especially to rural areas. The third is that doctors are too expensive. Utilization is seen as being "out of control," We should note that governments have not been really playing fair on this last issue. Although the structures and process of negotiating fee schedules have gradually been evolving from adversarial to more formalized "mutual accommodation" approaches[13] a number of these discussions have appeared to be more of a "take it or leave it" than a negotiation, and government has tended to take its ball and go home if it does not like the way a particular agreement ended up. A clear example is the ongoing saga of physician negotiations in Manitoba, and its "now you see it now you don't" binding arbitration. Ontario now has an agreement and joint management structure with the Ontario Medical Association (OMA), which includes caps based on physician earnings (rather than on patient needs). The cap kicks in at $400,000, and has affected about 5 percent of Ontario doctors. In exchange, the OMA got mandatory dues (the

Rand Formula), and is trying to decide whether it is a trade union or a professional body, and how it should be dealing with government. British Columbia has had acrimonious negotiations with physicians (including government decisions not to honour prior agreements). It has capped the aggregate increase in physician billings to 2 percent, and will claw back general practitioner billings over $300,000 and specialist billings over $360,000. Newfoundland froze physician fees and capped total Medicare funding. We expect this will get worse — both for doctors and in terms of unpleasantness — before it gets better.

In addition to these aggregate controls, provinces are paying considerable attention to such initiatives as guidelines and utilization management in their negotiations with physicians. This broadening of the focus of physician negotiations beyond increases to the fee schedule reflects a more general effort to manage health-care resources. This will be discussed as part of the sixth theme, *appropriateness*.

The fifth theme, however, is a *looming threat to national standards*. Universality, comprehensiveness, portability, and accessibility may all be threatened. In a paper for HEAL, Deber was rash enough to predict where she saw the likely trouble spots as federal control over Medicare declines. Erosion is most likely to begin with:

- imposition of "small" user fees and co-payments (e.g., Quebec's proposed $5 for an "unnecessary" emergency room visit)

- redefinition of "medically necessary" to allow the de-insurance of services, beginning with those "marginal" activities not strictly required under the terms of the *Canada Health Act* (i.e., that were not included in the *Hospital Insurance and Diagnostic Services Act* or the *Medical Care Act*)

- redefinition of eligibility requirements (e.g., to require payment of premiums before someone can be covered)

- limitations on portability, with restrictions on payment for out-of-province treatment, and

- an increased role for private insurers to pick up the areas vacated by Medicare.

These pressures are likely to be most severe on the poorest provinces. For example, Newfoundland is already spending a far greater percentage of its GDP to maintain a lower level of per capita spending than are the richer provinces. As these trends continue, the poorer provinces (particularly those in Atlantic Canada) may find it very difficult to maintain current programs without more federal money. In addition, these provinces are more dependent upon national activities in such areas as standard setting or policy guidelines, and less likely to have provincial resources available (let alone in place) to pick up these pieces. An optimistic possibility would see cooperative arrangements arising among provinces or regions, and a greater role for national associations in picking up some of those pieces (e.g., quality assessment, standard setting). A less optimistic one would find that certain activities (e.g., quality assurance, technology assessment, health information) would not get done at all there, or would get done on a shoestring.

In consequence, we believe that if current trends continue, the provincial plans are likely to diverge.

The sixth change is, we think, a hopeful one. It is a greater focus on why we are doing what we are doing, that is, on outcomes, and the *appropriateness* of care. There is considerable activity here, albeit still largely unconnected and at early stages. This theme assumes that we can maintain high-quality universal Medicare, if we make sure that service provision is more efficient and that services are only provided to those who are likely to benefit from them.

There are lots of buzzwords here. One is *utilization management*, especially in large hospitals. We are finally starting to get some use out of the clinical information systems that have been developed in the last decade, although there are still lots of data problems. (For example, there is considerable variation in how clinical events are documented, and reimbursing on the basis of diagnosis is likely to make this much worse.) One trend has been the emergence of "appropriateness screens" to identify patients who warrant further review (especially re: admission and discharge, but systems are also set up to enforce protocols).

There are some real risks here, and we are seeing them south of the border. Physicians and patients have largely lost control of care decisions, which are now made by insurance companies. In too many cases, they do not control costs, but just shift them elsewhere (often, to patients and their families). In other cases, they may encourage deception and other cynical practices to bypass utilization guidelines or to maximize reimbursement, or even to refuse to treat patients who are likely to be expensive. There is little information available on whether utilization management has helped to control costs, but it certainly seems to have aggravated physician-hospital relationships.[14]

More clinically credible are the efforts of professional bodies to develop guidelines of their own. These efforts are being made partly to protect professional influence, but also to ensure that we do not lose sight of quality in the impetus to control costs.[15] An important — and much missed — figure here was the late Adam Linton, who made a strong case for guidelines as a method of improving medical practice, and helped convince his colleagues in the OMA of their importance.[16] The Canadian Medical Association, the Association of Canadian Medical Colleges, provincial licensing bodies, and the Royal College of Physicians and Surgeons are working together on efforts to develop guidelines on guidelines, which encourage physician participation in developing them, and make sure the results are flexible enough and allow for continuing review. A number of contentious issues remain, including who should be responsible for developing guidelines, and how they should be used.

Another buzzword is Continuous Quality Improvement (CQI), also referred to as Total Quality Management (TQM). These concepts derive from quality management in industry. As Berwick has stated, the goal of these efforts is to shift emphasis from detecting "bad apples" towards improving the overall level of performance. Although the terms CQI and TQM have faddish overtones and have spawned a considerable consulting industry, the underlying concepts are critically important.

In effect, the appropriateness movement has two key goals. The first is to redesign direct care and support services to be more efficient and effective. An x-ray which must be repeated because the original is misplaced not only creates waste — it may actually harm the patient by exposing him or her to additional radiation. More broadly, quality improvement and other initiatives focused on appropriateness ask individual practitioners and health-care organizations to be more conscious of ensuring that "the right service is delivered by the right provider at the right time." Much remains to be done in developing the information management and health-care delivery systems capable of operationalizing these concepts. The goal, however, has been widely recognized and approved, most recently by the Canadian deputy ministers of health in formulating a vision for quality.[17]

The second goal of the appropriateness movement is to ensure that health-care services are not only "technically" excellent, but fulfill the needs of patients and communities. This in turn requires greater understanding of their needs. At the community level, there are some hopes that regional and participatory structures may improve community responsiveness. On the patient level, a key idea is patient empowerment [18] working on the assumptions that patients are the best guides of what they want and need. What happens when these two concepts collide (e.g., when patients want treatments which the community is unwilling to provide) has not yet been well thought through.

A Chinese curse is reputed to be "may you live in interesting times." We do. There are lots of ideas around. Some are zombies, and we would place the "de-insure/user fees/ we can't afford Medicare" arguments in that category. Others, however, have the potential to improve what is already an excellent system.[19] Unnecessary care is no bargain, however cheaply it is delivered, and enhanced partnership with patients is likely to be a good thing.

As can be seen by this cursory review of current activities, we are now charging forward. We can only hope that we are moving in the right direction.

Notes

This work was supported in part by Health and Welfare Canada, National Health Research and Development Program, Grant No. 6606-3007-63.

[1] Robert S. Evans, *Strained Mercy: The Economics of Canadian Health Care* (Toronto: Butterworths, 1984).

[2] Paul Starr, *The Meaning of Privatization,* project on the Federal Social Role, Working Paper 6 (Washington, DC: National Conference on Social Welfare, 1985).

[3] Raisa B. Deber, Orvill Adams, and Lynn Curry, "A typology of health-care systems" in preparation.

[4] Delivery, in general, has remained in the hands of the private sector, although the provincial government also chose public delivery for certain activities (particularly public health, psychiatric hospitals).

[5] Raisa B. Deber, *Regulatory and Administrative Options for Canada's Health Care System,* paper prepared for HEAL (The Health Action Lobby), Ottawa, 1 October 1991.

[6] See Douglas E. Angus, *Review of Significant Health Care Commissions and Task Forces in Canada Since 1983-84,* prepared for the CMA Canadian Nurses Association and Canadian Hospital Association, Ottawa, December, 1989; Douglas E. Angus, "A great Canadian prescription: Take two commissioned studies and call me in the morning" in Raisa B. Deber, Gail G. Thompson, (eds.), *Restructuring Canada's Health Services System: How Do We Get There From Here?* (Toronto: University of Toronto Press, 1992), pp. 49-62; and Sharmila L. Mhatre and Raisa B. Deber, "From equal access to health care to equitable access to *health*: A review of Canadian provincial health commissions and reports," *International Journal of Health Services*, 22(4), 1992: 645-668.

[7] Alistair Thompson, *Financing Health Care,* paper prepared for HEAL (The Health Action Lobby), Ottawa, 30 August 1991.

[8] Robert G. Evans, "U.S. influences in Canada: Can we prevent the spread of Kuru?" in Deber and Thompson, *Restructuring Canada's Health Services System,* pp. 143-148.

[9] Daniel M. Fox, and Howard Leichter, "Rationing care in Oregon: The new accountability," *Health Affairs* 10(2), 1991:7-27.

[10] Paul Gamble, "Hospital resources in Metropolitan Toronto: The reality versus the myth," in Deber and Thompson, *Restructuring Canada's Health Services System,* pp. 339-346.

[11] Ontario, Southwestern Ontario Comprehensive Health System Planning Commission (E. Orser, Chair), *Working Together to Achieve Better Health for All* (Toronto: Ontario Ministry of Health, 1991).

[12]Ontario, Steering Committee, Ontario Public Hospitals Act Review, *Into The Twenty-First Century: Ontario Public Hospitals* (Toronto: Ontario Ministry of Health, 1992).

[13]See Jonathan Lomas, Cathy Charles, Janet Greb, *The Price of Peace: The Structure and Process of Physician Fee Negotiations in Canada* Working Paper Series 92-17 (Hamilton, Ont.: McMaster University, Centre for Health Economics and Policy Analysis, 1992).

[14]B.G. Gray and M.J. Fields (eds.), *Controlling Costs and Changing Patient Care? The Role of Utilization Management* (Washington, DC: National Academy Press, 1989).

[15]See Donald Berwick, "Continuous improvement as an ideal in health care" *New England Journal of Medicine* 320 (1)1989:53-56, and *Curing Health Care* (San Francisco: Jossey Bass, 1990).

[16]A. Linton and D. Peachy, "Guidelines for medical practice: 1: The reasons why," *Canadian Medical Association Journal* 143 (6) 1990: 485-90.

[17]Canada, Working Group on Quality, *Toward a Vision for Quality in Health Care in Canada* (Ottawa: Conference of Deputy Ministers of Health, 1992).

[18]Raisa B. Deber, "Directing information to the patient," paper prepared for CHEPA.

[19]Mhatre and Deber, "From equal access to health-care to equitable access to *health*."

2

Review and Forecast of
Federal-Provincial Relations

Amelita A. Armit

In reflecting on my topic, "review and forecast of federal and provincial relations," I was reminded of the opening lines of Charles Dickens' *A Tale of Two Cities* —

> It was the best of times, it was the worst of times, it was the age of wisdom, it was the age of foolishness, it was the epoch of belief, it was the epoch of incredulity, it was the season of Light, it was the season of Darkness, it was the spring of hope, it was the winter of despair, we had everything before us, we had nothing before us, we were all going direct to Heaven, we were all going direct the other way.

This was a description of events in 1775, and I am sure you will agree with me that it does not take much poetic licence to use the same words to describe the feelings and perceptions of Canadians during the many stages of evolution of our health-care system. Think about the introduction of Medicare and the physicians strike in Saskatchewan; think about the uphill struggle for the *Canada Health Act* which ended extra-billing by doctors; think about our current policy context.

There is so much ferment in our health-care system today, as we adapt to new economic and social realities. I echo what many have said: our health-care system is at a crossroad; it is at the very same crossroad that sees us re-examining our values and defining our identity. And so we face difficult choices. And the road we take from here will be influenced by many factors, not the least of which is our unique branch of federal-provincial relations. Let me examine the dynamics of this interface and its impact on the evolution of our health-care policy by providing an historical sketch of where we have come from and where we are today by describing the major policy objectives during these periods and providing some observations on prospects for the future.

THE EARLY YEARS: THE QUEST FOR UNIVERSALITY

Our health-care system is best described as a set of 12 interlocking health insurance schemes linked to national standards at a federal level. This structure flows from our constitutional arrangement where health care is a matter of provincial jurisdiction. Federal involvement to a large extent comes from its exercise of its spending power and the general rubrics of pursuing good government and the national interest.

The seeds of our national health-care system came from the first innovation in Saskatchewan in 1947 when it introduced a public, universal hospital insurance scheme. This was followed by similar plans in British Columbia, Alberta and Newfoundland. The federal government subsequently enacted the *Hospital Insurance and Diagnostic Services (HIDS) Act* to encourage the development of hospital insurance programs in all provinces. This legislation enabled the federal government to share in the costs of provincial hospital insurance plans that met minimum eligibility and coverage standards. By 1961 all provinces and territories had plans providing comprehensive coverage for hospital care and covering 95 percent of the population. Thus began the principle of universality in our health system.

THE 1960s: UNIVERSALITY PLUS

The universal hospital insurance scheme was followed by the establishment of a complementary medical care plan. Once more the principle of universality was a key building block in the establishment of a national medical care program. Again with Saskatchewan leading the way in 1962 and spurred by the recommendations of the Royal Commission on Health Services (Hall Commission) in 1964, the federal government enacted the 1966 *Medical Care Act*. This enabled the federal government to enter into conditional cost-sharing arrangements — approximately a 50/50 basis — on provincial medical-care services. The "condition" essentially was adherence to certain standards which were to become the five principles that characterize our present health-care system: universal coverage; comprehensive service coverage, accessibility, portability of coverage; and public administration of insurance plans.

Provinces were quick in establishing medical-care insurance plans. By 1969 all ten provinces had a plan in place and by 1972, the territories had joined in and Canada's national health insurance system was in place.

THE 1970s: WHO'S IN CHARGE?

The funding arrangements embodied in the HIDS Act of 1957 and the *Medical Care Act* of 1966 gave the federal government a significant influence in shaping provincial-territorial health insurance plans. The cost-sharing arrangements produced a "steering effect" on provincial health expenditures. Because only hospital and medical services were eligible for federal funding, provinces' health spending were primarily on treatment and institution-based health services to maximize federal contributions. These fiscal arrangements cramped provincial directions, so to speak, and limited their flexibility to redirect resources to alternative community-based health services. This constraint became particularly problematic in the mid-to-late seventies as the community health service movement started to get a lot of attention as an alternative health delivery system. Provincial concerns with the cost-sharing arrangement were also centred on the federal scrutiny it entailed and its associated administrative and bureaucratic implications.

The federal government had its own set of concerns with the 1966 cost-sharing arrangement. Federal outlays were linked to provincial spending which were open-ended and unpredictable. This constrained the ability to plan and budget accordingly.

It was this mutual recognition of specific problems that paved the way for federal-provincial discussions that eventually culminated in the Established Programs Financing arrangements (EPF) in 1977. Under EPF, federal contributions to the provinces for three programs that were already established — hospital insurance, medical insurance and post-secondary education — were no longer based on actual provincial expenditures. Instead, federal contributions were in the form of a block fund transfer, with 1975-76 base year expenditures, escalated on the basis of population changes and GNP growth. An unconditional transfer for extended health-care services was also included in these arrangements.

EPF was a funding mechanism that sought to respect provincial jurisdiction in the management of the health delivery system and at the same time maintain national objectives in health financing. From a policy implementation perspective, EPF changed the nature of federal-provincial relations in health care. As the two levels of government began to operate more independently, their roles became more distinct. The federal government's role as a financier/banker gave it a low-key profile as provincial governments rightfully asserted their roles as managers of the health system.

The post-1977 period showed a flowering of provincial experimentation and innovation with delivery systems, for example, more community-based programs such as home care; and the expansion in the range and scope of services covered by provincial medical plans such as dental programs for children, drug plans for seniors, and prosthetics and other aids to daily living benefits. The flexibility afforded by EPF block funding, coupled with a relatively buoyant economy were significant factors that led to the mix of benefits and services that people have come to perceive as the components of our health-care system today.

THE 1980s: EARLY WARNING SIGNS OF REFORM

The tremendous growth in health-care programs in the late 1970s inevitably produced subsidiary effects in terms of increased demands and increased expectations from both the supply and the demand side of the health system. These pressures, in turn generated a host of health policy issues, the most prominent was the principle of accessibility, which was precipitated by the extra-billing/user-charge issue of the early 1980s.

The public debate on extra-billing by physicians was fought on many lines — ideology, politics, economics, and public administration. And through this debate the issue of convergence was the national character of Medicare and the principles behind it. The federal government took a prominent role in this debate as spokesman for the national interest and commissioned a series of reports and internal analyses.

The Hall Commission Report of 1980 concluded that the federal government had the responsibility to revise health insurance legislation to deal with extra-billing and user charges and to set objectives to reaffirm the national character of Medicare. The Breau Review of federal-provincial financing arrangements came to the same conclusion. Thus the role of guardian of Medicare was thrust squarely upon the shoulders of the federal government.

At the 1982 Conference of Federal-Provincial Health Ministers, federal Health Minister Monique Begin presented the federal government's proposals for revising existing health insurance legislation, including provisions to address extra-billing and user charges. This was the proposed *Canada Health Act (CHA)*. The provinces were opposed to any legislative change, despite their commitment to national principles including accessibility.

During the development of the *Canada Health Act,* the federal government and the provinces failed to find common ground despite repeated meetings. At both the political and official levels, relations were tense because the provinces resented federal "interference." The provinces also resented being "forced" to take on the medical associations in the provinces over the issue of extra-billing. Meanwhile, the federal government became increasingly impatient with the provincial lack of resolve. The result was an impasse in which differences could not be amicably resolved.

The conflict that existed between the two groups is illustrated by a statement issued by the Conference of Provincial Ministers of Health in September 1982. It said that the provincial ministers would consider a constitutional challenge to the authority of the federal government to proceed with the draft health insurance legislation based on current federal proposals. Further federal-provincial meetings failed to produce more constructive results.

By the Spring of 1983, the federal government was committed to new legislation for the purposes of clarifying the conditions; establishing provisions for enforcement; and improving accountability to Parliament for the expenditure of funds in respect of health-care services. In order to bring the federal views directly to the public and to various health professionals, the federal government carried out a publicity campaign centred around the policy paper, *Preserving Universal Medicare.*

The *Canada Health Act* was given first reading on December 1983 and given Royal Assent on 17 April 1984. Less than two weeks before this, a communiqué issued by the provincial and territorial ministers stated that the *Canada Health Act* was "being imposed over the objections of the provinces and territories."

The difficulties surrounding the passage of the CHA were not easily overcome. Federal-provincial relations were uncomfortable even while negotiations were undertaken regarding administrative issues and the proposed regulations. The situation remained tense especially until 1987 when the last of the refunds of federal withholdings with respect to extra-billing and user charges were made. The tension in relations necessitated a very low-key, non-confrontational approach on the part of the federal government.

Having said this, it should be noted that the CHA was accepted as a "fait accompli" by the provinces. The same cannot be said of the medical profession. The doctors had been as vocal in their dissent as the provinces. The Canadian Medical Association (CMA) and the Ontario Medical Association (OMA) launched a constitutional challenge of the *Canada Health Act.*

The turning point in federal-provincial relations did not come until the Spring of 1985 when the Federal-Provincial Conference of Ministers established a spirit of collaboration and laid the groundwork for a general understanding concerning the administration and operation of the Act. This culminated in the June 1985 letter from Health Minister Epp to his provincial counterparts affirming the federal objective to uphold the principles of the CHA. This letter, from a policy implementation perspective, served also as a signal for the bureaucracy to adopt a consensual conciliatory versus adversarial approach to the resolution of issues under the CHA and its regulations.

It is interesting to note that while the federal government adopted a relatively low profile on the Medicare front during this period, it adopted a very proactive stance in another important area of health policy — health promotion. Picking up on the themes of the 1974 Lalonde Report on *a New Perspective on the Health of Canadians*, it released in 1986 a *Framework on Health Promotion: Achieving Health for All*, which became a seminal influence to current national health promotion strategies. I am not sure whether this policy positioning on health promotion at this time was part of a deliberate strategy. In retrospect, the timing was excellent, especially when you look at the direction of the reforms proposed for health care in the late 1980s and the reforms proposed today.

The Late 1980s saw the return of health-care issues to the forefront of the public agenda. By this time, cost pressures in the system — from changing public needs and expectations to human resource issues — were becoming more apparent. These pressures were exacerbated by a weak economy and a tight fiscal framework. A spate of provincial task forces and commissions were undertaken during this period to look at future directions in health care. Many significant changes in health-care programming and delivery systems also occurred during this period, mostly centred on the issues of cost effectiveness, efficiency and accountability. For example, many provinces introduced measures to adapt their health systems to new realities: there was a definite decline in the expansion of health programs; there was capping of payments to physicians; hospital beds were closed; there was selective de-insurance or introduction of co-payments for non-medically necessary services. These changes or adjustments engendered a public perception of a health-care system in crisis. The public began to express openly and loudly its fear that the health-care system it had come to enjoy might not be there when needed.

These fears were magnified when the federal government amended the fiscal arrangements four times to limit the growth of EPF transfers to the provinces to address its own constrained fiscal framework and deficit. These actions by the federal government were seen not only by the provincial governments, but also by the general public as a retreat on the federal government's commitment to universal, accessible health care. It would seem that the public debate on the national character of the health-care system, on its underlying values and principles — the debate reminiscent of that preceding the passage of the *Canada Health Act* — would be resurrected all over again.

The public outcry was given further legitimacy as major stakeholders came out to present their positions to government and formed coalitions to galvanize government into action. One of these was the Health Action Lobby — HEAL — a coalition of seven major health organizations — the CMA, Canadian Nurses Association (CNA), Canadian Public Health Association (CPHA), Long-Term Care Association; Canadian Psychological Association and the Canadian Consumer Association. HEAL was one of the first groups to offer recommendations to governments on the substance and process for preserving the Medicare system. The significance of seven associations, with competing interests, coming together and speaking with one voice on the future of the health-care system was not lost on the federal government. Health care clearly is an issue right on top of the public policy agenda.

THE 1990s: NO EASY SOLUTIONS

Our review of the evolution of our health-care system, thus far, has shown that policy innovations were the by-products of intensive, often complex federal-provincial interactions. Many times the innovation started at the provincial level and most of the time, the enhancement and diffusion of that innovation was given a national character by the federal government. As we entered the 1990s, the national character of the health-care system was very much to the fore. Part of it was due to the constitutional discussions and the proposals to entrench the five principles of the CHA in a social charter. The other part of it stemmed from the momentum of significant changes and adjustments in practically all provincial health systems. There was a lot of talk about reforming the health-care system, not only in response to the fiscal conditions brought about by the deceleration in the rate of growth of federal fiscal transfers, but also in response to the growing public understanding of the need for a health system focused on "wellness" and the broad determinants of health. The problems and opportunities facing governments and society as a whole in this area were captured in the First Report of the Standing Committee on Health and Welfare, Social Affairs, Seniors and the Status of Women, entitled *The Health Care System in Canada and its Funding: No Easy Solutions*, tabled in the House of Commons on 21 June 1991. The issues identified in this report are still with us today and remains and will remain, the context for the health policy environment for the remainder of this decade.

How have federal and provincial governments responded to the challenges outlined in the Report? What are the prospects for the future? Let me offer *five key observations*.

First: There is an acknowledgement at the highest levels of public decision making on the need to act now to adapt and adjust our health-care system to new economic, social and political realities.

In September 1991, the federal and provincial ministers of health released the so-called "Winnipeg Statement," confirming their support for preserving the five principles of the CHA; recognizing the need to assure adequate funding to support the system and identifying key areas of action such as quality assurance, physicians resources planning, etc.

In March 1992, the first ministers directed the ministers of health and finance to meet and deal with issues related to the cost of the health-care system, the need to link the broad principles of the health system to the objectives of sustainability, affordability, flexibility and effectiveness of the system without destabilizing provincial, territorial and federal financing.

On 18 June 1992, the health and finance ministers met in Ottawa to act on the first ministers' directives. This is the first time in 25 years that these two groups of ministers have met, and there was an open and frank exchange of perspectives on the fiscal context and the steps taken by governments to manage the health system within this context.

Second: There is a consensus that the nature of the problems facing the health system requires collaborative action. In other words, the preservation of our health-care system is not a federal problem; it is not a provincial problem, but a *NATIONAL* problem. This implies concerted, coordinated and reinforcing actions and strategies at all levels of government. Partnership is a key operating principle. Again, if I may refer to the health and finance minister's meeting, the spirit invoking a national issue was very much at play. There was no finger-pointing; there was no "fed-bashing"; but rather a vigorous defence and explanation of various points of view, to achieve a common purpose: preserving our health system.

Third: There is agreement on the *direction* of health reform. The key objectives are cost-containment, effective management and redirection of the system from an emphasis on health care to a broader, more comprehensive and integrated view of health, emphasizing health promotion, prevention and healthy public policy.

Fourth: Key areas on the substance of policy and program reform, requiring national strategies, have been identified. Examples include the following:

1. Health Manpower Resource Planning — especially physician resources.

    A conference on physician resources was held on 22-23 June and was sponsored by the Ontario and federal governments to examine the issues and recommendations raised by the Barer-Stoddart Report. The conference stemmed from the January 1992 meeting of federal, provincial and territorial ministers of health when they agreed on a national strategy to manage physician resources. Key elements of the strategy include reducing medical school enrolments and post-graduate medical training positions, addressing the appropriate distribution of physician manpower; and the establishment of clinical practice guidelines, etc.

2. National strategy for quality in health care, focusing on variance-utilization rates; outcome indicators, appropriateness and effectiveness of services, etc.

3. National Health Information Strategy — through the proposed establishment of an Institute on Health Information.

Fifth: The circle for decision making is being widened. The reform of the health system is definitely being opened to include the participation of all stakeholders — providers, consumers, professional groups, and interest groups. A variety of mechanisms is being used to accomplish this, not just the traditional public consultations and meetings but also through structural measures such as decentralized decision making, regionalized funding and enhanced citizen participation, or membership in hospital and community boards.

A key aspect of broader citizen involvement in re-orienting the health-care system is the consensus among ministers of health, supported by the ministers of finance, of the need to launch a nation-wide strategy to inform Canadians about their roles and responsibilities in respect of receiving the most appropriate health-care services. Linked to this concept is the idea of managing our expectations from the system; learning more about how it works, what works and being active participants in decisions relating to personal health. The media, lately, have made significant strides in this area and we will begin to see a coordinated effort among governments to intensify this type of public information and education.

What then are the prospects for the future of our health-care system? I am very optimistic, having observed and heard the deliberations of finance and health ministers during their meetings. Finance ministers gained a deeper insight into the complexities of managing health-care systems and an appreciation of the efforts made by health ministers to contain costs and improve efficiency while maintaining high standards of care. Health ministers got the strong message that the fiscal framework must be maintained and they responded firmly, particularly to the federal government, that they must be assured of a stable and predictable funding base if they are to succeed in their reform efforts.

What we have seen and heard at these meeting is the beginning of an ongoing dialogue between the federal and provincial health and finance ministers on the interconnections between their respective agendas. While there was no specific agreement on another meeting date, I have no doubt that when the finance ministers meet to review fiscal transfers, the concerns of health ministers will be an important context for their deliberations. The recognition of this policy interdependence is a very important outcome of the meetings. This, together with another affirmation of the five principles of the *Canada Health Act* and the context of affordability within a defined fiscal framework, are very clear and strong directives for health policy reform.

The challenges are tremendous. The opportunities are also tremendous. I go back to paraphrasing Charles Dickens — there will be times of Light and times of Darkness during this period of transition. But it can be done — there are common values; there is a collective will; there is commitment; there are many good ideas; and there is a sound health-care system. All these things augur well for reform.

INNOVATION

3

Role of Continuous
Quality Improvement

W. John S. Marshall

The title of this paper has been arranged to suggest that health care faces a challenge, that innovations are required and that we need to try to assess what impact this particular innovation can have in meeting the challenge. To date, the experience in the United States and Canada with Continuous Quality Improvement (CQI) has been mainly recorded in the hospital sector. I suggest that the principles of this methodology can and must be applied much more broadly across the health-care sector.

First, the challenge. Are we really facing a challenge or is it all rhetoric. I am convinced that only if we agree and truly understand the nature of the challenge that faces us can we energize people to make the necessary changes that will allow us some possibility of meeting that challenge. In this paper I shall mention four facets that suggest that the areas in the next decade or two where the stresses and challenges of the health-care industry are going to expand exponentially.

First, simply, the same money is no longer going to be available. The balmy days of the 1960s and 1970s are over. The hedonistic lifestyle of the yuppy eighties when we thought we could ignore our problems and our past, and the realities of the nineties are upon us (dinks to dunks — double income no kids to double unemployment no kids).

The debt burdens that we are elevating for future generations are clearly intolerable and cannot continue. Governments and, indeed, the people they represent will no longer be prepared to foot the kinds of bills that the health-care industry has been imposing on them. It would be nice to think that our present problems in 1992 were only to do with a recession. In fact, they are simply that governments and the people are reaching the reality that we can no longer continue to increase spending. Quite simply, there will be less money paid to providers regardless of the amount of work they are being asked to do. While this could simply be met by cries of unfairness, it is certainly a challenge and one which, hopefully, will be met by some constructive alterations in the way in which providers react within the whole health-care system.

The second part of the challenge that we face is the aging of the population. Canada, to date, has *not* really begun to see the effect of the baby boom on its health-care industry. We were somewhat slower to react to the opportunities of the postwar period and are, as a result, a relatively late baby-booming country. But, it is not only the number of older patients that offers the challenge, there has been a dramatic increase year by year in the utilization of services by the older section of the population. A study undertaken for the Scott Task Force by Drs. Denton and Spencer, using HMRI database figures between 1980 and 1990, demonstrated that in spite of the relatively modest increase of the proportion of patients over 65 years old in the population from 9.7 percent to 12.4 percent, their bed utilization in acute care hospitals had risen from 33.9 percent to 44.5 percent over the decade.

However, this fact pales into relative insignificance when one looks at what has been happening to those over 75. This group, which represents less than 5 percent of the population, now consumes over one-quarter of all bed days used in acute care hospitals and I should point out that this occurred in spite of a significant reduction over the last few years in the length of stay of these patients. However, their rates of admissions and incidence of in-hospital care continue to rise dramatically year over year. This would have produced a crisis situation now had not both rates of admission and lengths of stay of all other groups fallen dramatically.

But make no mistake, the crisis is coming because the combination of increasingly limited economic resources, increased institutional use by the elderly and the prospect of the baby boom generation reaching the elderly group in a decade or so, suggests to me a sports car with a blind driver accelerating rapidly towards a brick wall.

The standard modern response to predicted disaster is that technology will offer an exit. In this case, however, technological innovation is the foot on the accelerator of the car that I have envisaged.

It is the success of technology that increases the costs of health care for the elderly. Both simple measures such as antibiotics and more complex interventions such as coronary artery by-pass grafts, renal dialysis, cardiac pacemaker vascular reconstructive surgery and cancer chemotherapy ensure the survival of patients with chronic degenerative disease in the status of permanent users of illness care.

The rate of technological innovation is increasing exponentially. Within one year the genetically engineered drug erythropoiten became the number one drug as far as cost is concerned in our hospital although limited to only 65 patients. The liberations of the use of this drug and the potential introduction of other mega-cost genetically engineered drugs exemplify the escalating cost of technology which is accelerating our juggernaut to its wall of destruction.

I would suggest that anyone who questions that there might be a challenge should now be somewhat convinced that the challenge is real and, indeed, is somewhat daunting.

WHAT IS CONTINUOUS QUALITY IMPROVEMENT?

The question that I will now attempt to address is in what way can the innovation of Continuous Quality Improvement (CQI) have an impact on the challenge faced in health care. My focus will be hospitals, but hopefully applicable to the whole system. What I want to do in addressing CQI is to outline the essential elements that lie behind this concept and to make some relatively bold assertions as to the applications of such concepts if they are to have an impact on the challenge we face.

I will not try, and indeed I am not qualified to give you a blueprint of the methods, strategy, tools and educational program that are required to lead an organization to a continuous improvement method of operation.

I do wish, however, to achieve a common understanding of the philosophical and practical bases on which CQI is founded, then to give a simple example of what it can do, and to make some bold assertions on what is really required if it is to contribute to our meeting the challenges.

The Definition

The definition I give here of Continuous Quality Improvement is not original, but it is mine. It is not original in that each word or phrase is taken from the writing of others, but it is mine in that they are arranged to suit my argument.

"Continuous Quality Improvement" is an explicit fact-based process in which the identified needs of the customers are understood and served by processes with the smallest possible variation leading to the most effective, achievable outcomes. Improvement occurs by continuous analysis of inputs, outcomes and processes by all those involved using specific tools resulting in changes being instituted and the processes being reanalyzed.

This is quite a mouthful, but I hope to be able to demonstrate the importance of each part of this definition.

Please note that apart from the words "Continuous Quality Improvement," I do not use the word "Quality" in the definition. We all have, I think, the idea that we know what the phrase "Quality of Care" means. However, when we attempt to define that idea, we become remarkably inept. At a recent meeting of the Patient Care Committee of our Board of Governors, we spent over an hour trying to reach a definition of the quality of patient care and, quite frankly, we failed.

Thinking about it, it became clear to me that no one around the table had any problem with the concept of the individual qualities of care, but it was the combination of multiple important qualities that could not be defined with any ease or any degree of unanimity. Thus, if I take a single admission for a spinal fusion, the quality of that episode of care cannot be defined only by the outcome, i.e., that the spinal fusion is solid; because many other factors contribute to the quality, the appropriateness of the decision to fuse, the admission process, the anaesthetic process, the nature and sterility of the operative procedure, the attitude and concern of the nursing staff, the nature of the follow-up, the communication with the family physician, not to mention the thousand other issues that support each activity mentioned. The fusion may, indeed, be solid but the patient may have spent three months in hospital with an infection, may have hated the food and may not have needed the operation in the first place so the outcome as the sole measure of quality is clearly inadequate.

Because of our difficulty in defining overall quality we must be careful not to use a single quality as a convenient surrogate for the total quality of care.

I had no difficulty in understanding the role of individual quality contributing to total excellence, but I had much greater difficulty in finding a general definition of a quality that would apply uniformly to all these individual qualities until I came across this definition in Kaizen, simply put, "A quality is anything that can be improved."

Its simplicity and relevance to the process of CQI form a philosophical bedrock on which I can rest the whole concept of continuous quality improvement. Thus, the overall quality of an episode of care, or a process of management or production, is made up of the sum of individual qualities that are individually identified as any aspect of that process or episode that can be improved.

It takes no great stretch of the imagination to see the limitless possibilities for improvement at every point in the complex process of delivering health care.

THE PROCESS

Using my definition of CQI as a base, I now examine features that can be identified in that definition and try to give some idea of the change and, indeed, paradigm shift that is required to see a continuous quality improvement environment work.

Explicit

It is vital that the needs of the customer or patient are identified explicitly at the outset. It is really somewhat terrifying how often professional and management decisions rely on implicit standards alone. There is no determination that other parties to the decision understand or agree with these standards or decisions.

The realization that it took the Supreme Court of Canada to define a doctrine of informed consent certainly suggests to me that many of the decisions taken on behalf and for patients were implicit rather than explicit. I am not sure that the Supreme Court has made a lot of difference.

In my neurosurgical practice, more often than not, patients referred to me would be unaware of what the nature of my specialty was or why they were seeing me. This immediately posed the danger that I would try to meet their referring physician's needs rather than theirs.

Kingston General Hospital has a neurosurgical spinal disc clinic set up to deal with patients with acute spinal problems suitable for surgery. Referring physicians knew the nature of this clinic and the purpose for its existence. However, at the time of their first appointment, 70 percent of patients had no knowledge that they were going to see a surgeon, nor had their primary care referring physicians mentioned that surgery was an option. One-half of those patients, when asked whether they would consider surgery said that they did not wish to, but it was clear that there were a significant number of those who were willing to accept surgery subsequently, but that willingness was based on the circumstance in which they found themselves at that clinic. The lack of explicitness clearly undermined the whole process in which the patients were able to choose the type of care available to them.

Being explicit means that not only must the customers'or patients' criteria be explicitly defined, but so must the professional criteria and standards be stated so that they can be examined and be subject to modification and improvement. It goes without saying that both these specific approaches to the patient's criteria and expectations, and the professional criteria and expectations will tend to expose misunderstandings.

Customer Focused

The continuous quality improvement environment is customer focused in that it is founded on the understanding that a service is being offered and that the customer — the one receiving the service — is the one who knows what is required. The explicit nature of the interaction between the customer and the provider mentioned above is the only way individual services can be customer centred. Outside specific interactions it is essential that the customers, in general, be consulted.

I must digress here for the moment because the word "customer" upsets many physicians, and I used to be one of them! I had always felt that "patient" was a sacred word and that whereas a "client" referred to someone you had a contract with, a patient was someone you had a responsibility to. Indeed I still do feel that way but as I came to understand the CQI paradigm, I realize that I had responsibilities to many people who were not my patients such as referring physicians, patients' relatives, nurses, orderlies, secretaries, etc.

I then accepted that perhaps the idea of a customer could also be someone with whom one had a responsibility to and that the patient was just a particular kind of customer within a specific medical professional paradigm. Thus I can now accept that the patient is, in fact, a customer. This, I suspect, is still difficult for some of my colleagues, but I think it is essential that a wider view of who our customers are is accepted.

The customer concept is important because it is vital that we recognize that we have internal and external customers and that a physician, for instance, has many customers other than patients. It must be recognized that there is an equality of interest between internal and external customers. Physicians cannot serve their external customers adequately unless they simultaneously serve their internal customers. An important point about customer centring is that each individual episode of care may involve different customers and, indeed, in one part of a relationship an individual may be the customer and in another part of the same relationship may be the provider.

For instance, in the functioning of an operating room, the operating room booking system serves me, the surgeon, by producing an orderly and appropriate list which, in turn, helps and assists the nursing staff to have the appropriate instruments and the appropriate patient there at the appropriate time. However, in making that system work, I serve the operating booking system by giving that system the appropriate information about my patients and my intentions in an appropriately and timely fashion so that the system can subsequently serve me.

The understanding of this mutually dependent customer-provider relationship is one that will serve to remove the arrogant inattention from many parts of our medical care bureaucratic system. Customer centring gives an opportunity to substitute mutually dependent cooperation for externally applied discipline and sanctions.

Process Oriented

At the centre of CQI is the notion that all productive work is based on processes and that workers rely on processes. It is relatively simple and easy to conceptualize the process in manufacturing a widget or an automobile, but it is much more difficult to conceptualize the process involved in setting up an acute trauma care service. However, the same combination of customers, workers, processes and supplies exists in this activity as in manufacturing a widget. The same methods can be used to analyze both sets of processes.

It must be understood that processes, not people, produce problems. CQI starts with the philosophy that people want to do good work, that they are motivated, that they want to be consistent and that they do not wish to be responsible for variation. The reason that people fall short of this ideal is because the processes supporting their work are flawed. Processes can be defined, analyzed and improved. People can be exhorted, rebuked, disciplined or fired. There is little doubt which is most productive.

Blaming the person without understanding the process is simultaneously to cause resentment and to prevent improvement. Understanding and improving the process without blaming the person simultaneously allows for process improvement and insightful performance improvement by the person involved.

In looking at processes it is essential that those processes central to the operation and those that have the most affect on its productivity are studied first. It is not possible to attack all processes at once and if this is attempted, overwhelming data, confusion, inertia and failure will result.

Initiating study of one process sets the system in motion because the analysis, data collection and improvement strategies for one process nearly always result in the identification of many other processes that require study and improvement. By being process focused, CQI is self-directed and self-stimulated.

Fact Based

Improvement of a quality cannot be achieved unless it can be measured. In the same way that scientific medicine is based on the assembly of facts and diagnostic tests which, when analyzed, form the basis for diagnostic and treatment planning. The management process of continuous improvement is no different when applied to industrial or medical processes. The essential element that must serve both processes are facts, data and measurements that measure all aspects of the process starting with the customers' needs and expectations, the parameters of the processes used, the nature and methods by which results are achieved and some measurement of the outcome so that they can be compared and improvements identified.

In the health-care industry we certainly do not lack data — we almost certainly do lack the correct data presented in the correct way. To start the process we must recognize and utilize the data we have and see if it could be presented in ways that are meaningful, or measuring the processes we wish to study.

For example, the data presently being collected by a budget department to report day surgery rates for funding by the ministry can be taken and analyzed to discover variations in the use of day surgery among disciplines and individuals. The study of these variations can improve the rate of surgical day care. Thus the budget department data can serve patient care improvement.

It is equally important that customer surveys, which have been traditionally carried out to give reassurance as to the standards of care being offered, are developed with a view to identifying processes that require study. This takes specific survey design.

It may also be that specific processes that we come across in our quest for improvement do not have a database that is applicable to them and we may have to set out to acquire data for individual specific processes. It is clear, however, that no realistic efforts to improve our performance in any sphere — be it clinical, administrative or even housekeeping — can be achieved without actually having valid measurements of that performance.

The process of CQI must be *variation centred*. The essence of ensuring improvement of any process is to identify the variations in that process and to make an attempt to limit them.

In a paper entitled "Controlling Variations in Health Care," Don Berwick introduced the medical community to the works of Walter Shewart, the father of quality process engineering, and made the plea that this statistical methodology developed by Shewart be applied to the variations in medical processes.

Processes can be defined as having two types of variations: those that are unintended and those that are intended. Unintended variations are the overwhelming cause of spending without demonstrated benefit. The removal of unintended variations would be one of the major steps to meeting the challenge that was outlined in the beginning. Shewart divided unintended variations into two types: common cause variations and assignable cause variations.

The first or common cause variations are those variations that may arise from a multiplicity of reasons but which, in the mass, are sufficiently organized and predictable such that they can be defined by a statistical process to fall within an expected range. Some people may describe this as the noise in the system. These variations are inherent in any process and the amount of variation clearly increases with the complexity of the process. They are, however, predictable and should not produce alarms or excessive reaction when they occur. Such reaction may be wasteful. However, if they are extremely large it suggests that basic features of the process may require adjustment.

More destructive, however, are the variations that Shewart described as assignable cause variations. They fall outside any statistical prediction and they represent the most disruptive events, and produce excessive and unproductive reactions. If such variations are unanalyzed and allowed to persist, the system becomes so noise-ridden that it is impossible to set any real parameters or expectations and a general laissez-faire attitude towards improvement is bound to occur.

Thus, it is essential that in studying any process statistical methods are used to identify the limits of common cause variations so that the disruptive assignable variations can be recognized, analyzed and eliminated. Only by doing so can one see whether the residual variation is of sufficient size to warrant total redesign of the process. For instance, lab tests will have a certain amount of variation that is based on the nature of the machinery, the nature of the chemical reagents that are used and perhaps, to some extent, the variation inherent in the human operator.

This may produce a variation that on a single sample is, say, 5 percent. However, should a reagent be improperly diluted by half, the resulting variation would be so massive as clearly to fall outside the statistical boundaries and would be an assignable variation.

Once the error that allowed the dilution is eliminated, one can examine whether or not the variation in the test quality of 5 percent is acceptable, or whether by changing the reagents, machinery or operator procedures, it can, say, be reduced to 2 percent.

This is systematic and simple industrial quality control and can be applied to the health-care delivery and decision making in a much broader scale. It is therefore very clear that if we are going to make improvements we must first look at the assignable cause or wide variations so that we can see the remaining noise in the system that can be subsequently addressed.

Then there are the intended variations. It seems intuitively reasonable that individual physician practices show some originality and variation; that surgeons use their own particular instruments; and that physicians may prefer a particular antibiotic.

But if the cost and non-value added work of these intended variations are not assessed, they become systemic, embedded, costly and useless. They all require examination and justification. This is a somewhat scary thought for physicians.

And, finally, there is what might be called policy variations. We have agreed that the transfer of health-care information is vital to the process of patient care, but we have also decreed that health-care records and x-rays belong to institutions. This results in repeated tests and x-rays causing risk to the patient and cost to the system. There are many other examples of conflicting funding and conflicting policies that could be addressed using a continuous quality improvement approach.

Cross Functional

Few health-care providers believe that they can act as solo professionals in the delivery of health care. However, when one examines most quality assurance programs in typical hospitals they have remained the jealously guarded purview of individual professional groups. Since the focus of these activities is people, not processes, and the bad apple approach dominates, this professional protectionism is only to be expected.

However, in a team environment the results of such personal protectionism are clear. First, there is a lack of understanding of the role of others in the processes. Second, there is a lack of ability to affect more than a small part of the process being studied and, finally, the distinct possibilities of mutually destructive changes by different professional groups simultaneously, but separately. It is thus clear that any process of continuous improvement must include all those involved in the process.

The results of such a change induce in all involved an awareness of the role of others which immediately raises the potential for problem solving and an understanding of the roles of other disciplines as they relate to and support the process under study.

This may seem like a simple, straight forward idea. However, let me assure you, it is a revolution in most of our thinking. This means that individual workers are made responsible for change. This means that medical practices are open to discussion by nurses and nursing practices by physicians, and both types of practices by orderlies. While this will be difficult to begin with it is the only way in which a true CQI environment can be developed.

Specific Tools

CQI comes with specific tools and methods. Indeed, this fact has the potential for exciting the interest and catching the attention of physicians more than any other. The basis of CQI is a problem-solving milieu that involves problem identification, analysis, solution design and checking the performance. Basically, it is the clinical, medical model to which every physician was brought up in medical school.

History taking, physical examination, diagnostic hypothesis, laboratory and radiological testing, diagnosis treatment planning, therapy and follow-up are the tools of clinical medicine. Customer surveys, process diagrams, cause and effect diagrams, pareto analysis, scatter plots and control diagrams are the tools of process analysis, an improvement developed for industrial processes. They are just as applicable to the processes of health-care delivery as they are to industry.

However, probably the most important point about these tools is that they are not the purview of a few individual experts. If the CQI environment is to be successful, these tools must be taught to everybody in the organization. They are relatively simple to use and can be a powerful tool in anyone's hand. Thus, the basic message is that when embarking on a CQI journey, education across the organization at every level is essential. Increasing the use of these tools in small, almost self-generating groups will completely change the ability of an organization to improve itself.

The final point of my definition of CQI is *continuous*. Once a single process has been studied, problems diagnosed, solutions found and put in place, then the results of implementation are checked and monitored to hold the gains. But that is not the end of the line for that particular process. Just because one part of the process has been improved does not mean all problems related to that process have been identified and that all possibilities for improvement in it have been addressed. It is clear that with an informed and educated work force other potential improvements in that particular process will be identified and can be addressed.

As a result of examining one process the related processes will have been brought to the attention of the team responsible. They can, in turn, be tackled. The cascade of process improvement efforts which can result is endless. Wasteful variation surrounds all those who can see it.

I have tried to outline the essential elements of CQI, but I have not, perhaps, adequately emphasized that the CQI environment means a philosophical and organizational change. It does, in essence, turn workers from doers and followers into thinkers and planners. It turns managers from commanders and disciplinarians into leaders, educators and servants. That sort of philosophical change cannot occur overnight and full implementation of a CQI environment is probably a five-to-ten-year project.

Can something occur in the meantime? Can the principles and tools of CQI be used before that environment is put in place? The answer is a resounding "yes"! I just want to give you one single example that occurred in the Kingston General Hospital during the time we were investigating the possibilities of CQI and before we had taken any steps really to introduce or apply the philosophy. However, this example used the tools and many of the principles of CQI and I think demonstrates the dividends that can be achieved.

When we started a really aggressive bed utilization drive involving the medical staff we wished to use HMRI data in order to press the urgency of the problem. We wanted to use current data, as physicians would continually tell us that "Oh, you're telling me what I did last year, I've changed."

We could not do it. We discovered that it took us up to 305 days from the time of discharge to submit records to HMRI. That meant that the hospital was missing HMRI deadlines, was not being included in comparative reports and we had little credibility with the medical staff in discussing utilization data. We were deprived of a major tool in looking for improvements.

The utilization management committee of the hospital met with the medical records department and suggested that an analysis of this problem might be worthwhile and, following that, the medical records department set out on its own improvement journey. I do not intend to detail the methods used but they basically included all the principles that I have annunciated. Two years later the situation has dramatically changed.

In April 1990 we needed 305 days for completion and submission of records. In March 1992 we only took 57 days! I am told that for April we are now down to 45 days. We achieved our primary objective. At the same time, we put our information on-line in the hospital which better addressed our internal utilization needs. So we have improved HMRI submission but, at the same time, we can use and analyze the data in-house prior to HMRI comparative reports.

At what cost was this done? The impressive thing is that in spite of processing the same number of discharges, and achieving six months more chart completion, the paid hours of the highest cost staff in the department, Health Records Analysts (HRAs) and Health Records Technicians (HRTs), dropped by 32 percent. Overtime dropped from 800 hours to 25 hours, and sick times as a proportion of paid hours, dropped from 4.5 percent to 1.8 percent. This demonstrates a massive increase in the morale of the department.

If this was all it would be sufficient praise for this quality improvement effort, but there have been other dividends. When this effort started there was seven feet of unfiled paper in the medical records department every single day. Now, at the end of each working day, there are no unfiled papers. Missing paper at follow-up appointments caused delays, staff were harassed, patients kept waiting. Typing of operating room reports and discharge summaries were back-logged up to two weeks, chart requests for quality assurance and medical research went unanswered.

All that is now gone. Charts are complete, available, dictation is so complete that stenos are available for other tasks in the department. The department has sufficient time to spread its improvement effort to educating physicians in chart completion practices that better serve coding and the Case Mix Group (CMG) assignment.

During a recent conversation with the director of the medical records department, it became clear to me that she now sees her staff as thinkers and planners, not followers and doers, and they see themselves in that light as well. But she was also aware that as she continues to pursue this improvement process in her own department, she is coming across barriers in other departments who have not yet begun the quality improvement journey, and the absolute necessity of cross functional institution-wide involvement has become clear.

This, I think, is a very simple and straightforward example of the power in a health-care institution of the principles of CQI; and if repeated across the institution the possibilities are obvious.

This example along with many of the others that are available in the literature particularly those from the national demonstration project, have concentrated to date on the supportive and service activities of hospitals and other institutions. Departments such as medical records, admission and discharge functioning processes in the emergency department, and processes in the laboratories, have been the major focus. Only very rarely have projects begun to touch at the fringe of the real heart of the medical process, clinical management and the processes within clinical management.

THE IMPACT OF CQI

I now come to my final question. Can the innovation of CQI make a significant and meaningful impact on the challenges facing health care?

There is no doubt that the example I have used of medical records, if used many times within the support and service systems of hospitals, can go a long way towards meeting the challenges resulting from the present fiscal restraint, and if this restraint were to continue, CQI applied to more and more support and service functions in the hospital would go a long way towards meeting that part of the challenge.

However, when I view the real nature of the challenge in the future from the increasing technology and increasing age and expectations of the population, it is inconceivable that merely nibbling around the edges by limiting the focus of CQI to supporting services can make any significant impact on that challenge.

It is essential that if CQI is to have the required impact, its role must expand to embrace the central issues that consume health-care resources, clinical care, clinical decision making and the processes that support them.

I am always somewhat nervous as a physician that I will be thought of as arrogant when I say that without the cooperation of physicians it is unlikely that the system can be saved. However, it is naive and short-sighted to the point of blindness, not to admit that it is largely the decisions of physicians and other clinical professionals that drive the standards, produce the demands and consume the bulk of resources, certainly in the illness care sector. Fiddling with the compensation models, changing inducements, capping incomes will, again, only play around the fringes of these issues. If unintended variations and poor processes in the medical records department waste money, the same defects in clinical decision-making processes are, to use Don Berwick's words, "robbing the health care system blind."

Can we apply the principles and practices of CQI to the clinical area? Will there not be physician resistance? Yes, certainly, there will be physician resistance. Can it be ever overcome? Yes, certainly, it can be overcome.

High quality patient care is an explicit, scientifically-based process in which the identified needs of the patient are understood and addressed by diagnostic and therapeutic processes with the smallest possible variation leading to the most effective resolution of the patient's problem. Improvement occurs by continuous scientific analysis of indications, processes of diagnosis and treatment, and of outcomes by all those involved using tools of problem solving and the scientific method resulting in changes in protocols being instituted and being reanalyzed.

This definition is one that I think could be accepted by all physicians. As you can see it is, in fact, the definition of continuous quality improvement.

So if medical records technicians can accept the process, so can physicians. However, this is a change and it is, indeed, a profound change. It is a change in viewpoint, it is a change in attitude that will require change in behaviour. Implementing the change from people-centred analysis to process-centred analysis and moving from professionally-centred activities to cross-functional activities will be very difficult and wrenching for some professionals. We truly are old dogs and these are truly new tricks.

CONCLUSION

Finally, I want to emphasize that CQI is not simply a technique. It is as much a paradigm shift as the Flexner revolution was 80 years ago. It is an umbrella under which our activities in health care can carry one, and if they follow the philosophical principles of CQI, they can yield spectacular dividends.

I get somewhat irritated with diagrams and statements that quality improvement is not compatible with quality assurance. Certainly, in so far as traditional quality assurance (QA) programs tend to be opinion-based, people-centred and professionally focused, they clearly do not fit within the CQI paradigm, but modern QA can, in fact, follow the principles of CQI. The presence of a CQI philosophy does not obviate the need for an institution to explicitly demonstrate its focus on quality, and assure that quality issues are being addressed.

This is quality assurance albeit carried out in the quality improvement paradigm. What then of all the other initiatives that are important today?

Indicator development, clinical guidelines, technology assessment, outcome studies, care plans, risk management, utilization management, computer-based professional expert systems and quality assurance. Where do they fit with CQI?

As I said, CQI is an umbrella. All these current trends and techniques can fit under the umbrella of CQI as long as they follow the basic supporting principle struts of CQI. If they tear away these protecting struts, the umbrella will collapse and they will be washed away in the deluge.

For example, if quality assurance is usurped by regulatory bodies which set minimal standards and seek people at fault, not processes, its failure is inevitable. If outcome research becomes professionally focused, not patient focused, little can be expected of it, and if technology assessment is left in the hands of single discipline interest groups, not cross functional teams, no real progress will be made. If indicators do not address processes they are useless. If utilization managers fail to assist physicians in changing practices, but merely chastise them, they will be resisted. If planned development does not involve all members of the team such plans will be rejected.

If risk management merely addresses legal costs and fails to improve processes, little good will result. But, if the message is taken, there is no doubt in my mind that CQI can have a major impact on the challenge we face. But this will only happen if the conversion that has started in the institution spreads through the system, and the supports of the CQI umbrella are kept in place and are applied to all our innovations.

The paradigm shift is here. If it is not recognized the system will fail. If it is recognized, at least we have some chance of meeting the challenges we face.

4

The Health Encounter Card Pilot Project: An Innovation in Health Care

Christel A. Woodward and Lynn Curry

In the past decade, rapid development has occurred in computer readable card technology which has promise for applications in the health-care field. Particularly smart cards, which are credit-card-sized plastic devices that contain microscopic integrated electronic circuits, can provide the user with both a secure method of storing and carrying personal information and with a way to access resources in a network of computers.[1] The integrated circuit chips contained in smart cards can perform the functions of a microprocessor, memory and an input/output interface. They can be carried in the same way that individuals now often carry the magnetic stripe credit cards issued by financial institutions. However, they can store significantly more information and offer more security to users.

The smart card, applied to health care, holds the promise of being a portable patient record and providing an important way of managing and communicating health information. The smart card might carry the individual's health history (e.g., major illnesses, injuries, operations, chronic conditions), information about preventive health (immunization status and date, date and type of last preventive health screenings, etc.) as well as information about use in medical emergencies (e.g., blood type, drug and other sensitivities, current medications). The card could be read by health professionals working with the patient on a need-to-know basis. Information on the health smart card would be updated during each encounter of the health service to provide information on recent encounters with health professionals, medications received and diagnostic and therapeutic procedures performed.

Although Europe has led the way in the development and application of smart card technology to the health-care field, several studies of the use of smart card technology in health-care applications are occurring currently in Canada.[2] One project in North Bay, Ontario examined the application of the technology in community pharmacies. Over 500 veterans who received prescription drug benefits paid for by Veterans Affairs, Canada were involved in the evaluation of the card acceptance and potential benefits of the technology in capturing a medication history and current prescriptions.[3] Another project is currently underway at Laval University's community health department while a third project involving Lions Gate Hospital and a group of physicians in North Vancouver is currently being planned.[4] Greenshield Prepaid Services has also begun a larger pilot project in Essex County, Ontario to test a smart card application to monitor medications. In contrast to the earlier project in North Bay, this project involves about 12,000 consumers. Some physicians and the emergency department of a local hospital will be equipped with reader work stations as well as participating pharmacists.

This paper describes a project initiated by the Ontario Ministry of Health (MOH) to examine the feasibility of using smart card technology as a personal health card which would capture all health-care encounters. It highlights the rationale for the project, its development and proposed implementation, and the focus and features of its evaluation.

RATIONALE FOR THE ENCOUNTER CARD PROJECT

During the 1980s, it became apparent that the information systems of the MOH, initially designed in the early 1970s to administer the newly introduced universal health insurance plan, were not readily amendable for the changing expectations of the role and goals of the health-care system in Ontario. Several commissions and task forces [5] created by the MOH produced reports that called for a stronger role by individual consumers in health and health-care matters, greater integration of the health-care delivery system and a more active management of the health-care system in partnership between the MOH and the health professionals. The Spasoff Report explicitly set as a goal "That Ontario health data be improved, beginning with an expansion of routinely collected databases to render them useful for planning and evaluation."

In response to these reports, the MOH began planning for the redevelopment of its systems to provide better information for management and planning of health care.[6] This initiative was part of the planning for increased leadership in reshaping the health-care system to meet the explicit goals set.

Of particular concern was that computerized information systems for many MOH funded programs had been developed separately to meet the particular needs of the program developed (e.g., home care, OHIP, air ambulance services, health unit immunization programs, etc.). They tended to have somewhat different data elements and used different coding schemes. The information collected was defined mainly by the way the program was funded. Data acquisition from programs is often slow. Total services by individuals across programs cannot be readily tracked and different programs cannot be compared because data are not comparable across programs.[7]

A first step in the re-development of the MOH's data systems involved issuing unique health numbers to each resident of Ontario and this was accomplished in 1990-91. The second stage involved thinking through and assessing the feasibility of collecting comparable timely information about patients' encounters with the health-care systems across health-care providers and settings. The health encounter card pilot project emerged as a vehicle for discussion with health professionals, hospitals and other health-care agencies about what information can and should reasonably be gathered about patients' encounters with the health-care delivery system that would aid management and planning in the health-care system.

The choice of a health encounter smart card pilot project had a broader rationale than simply being a method to allow dialogue with health professionals and agencies about information needs for management and planning for health care. Hospitals and providers were beginning to adopt computer technology to manage their own information needs and this trend is likely to increase rapidly. The MOH saw that a window of opportunity existed to define some basic, core elements of such computerized information systems (and their coding schema) before so many different information systems emerged that it would be difficult to obtain comparable information across sites and programs. Ideally, the data sent to the MOH would be a subset of routine data collected by each provider or facility. Further, using smart card technology held promise for meeting another major goal: empowering individuals by providing them with more information about their health and health care. Each individual would have ready access to information about their health and treatment of their health problems. Timelines of data retrieval might also be enhanced by the electronic transmission of encounter data at or near the time of the encounter to the MOH if the technology was feasible and acceptable to patients and providers. Use of health encounter cards also holds the promise that, by improving communication between the patient and providers and among relevant providers about investigations done and treatment provided, redundancies and gaps in the management of health-care problems could be reduced and quality of care improved. The health encounter card project was developed to assess whether the potential of the card could be realized in practice.

Perceived Potential Benefits of a Health Encounter Card System

In planning for the health encounter card project, the project team tried to identify all of the benefits that the encounter card might provide to various interested and affected parties. Although not all of these potential benefits can be explored in the initial pilot project which has a more limited scope of objectives, they buttress the importance of initiating the first stage of evaluation of the health encounter card.

Consumers. A health encounter card system has the potential to strengthen the role of individuals in their health and health care. Currently, health-care consumers lack a convenient, accurate, up-to-date record of their health problems and the care that they have been receiving. They are often asked repeatedly to describe problems that they are experiencing and the care that has been provided to them. Many of the same background questions will be asked by each provider whom they encounter, sometimes within the same clinic, the same hospital and certainly between different types of providers. Unfortunately, both because the care received is not accurately recalled or is not fully understood, many consumers have a less than complete awareness of the health care that they have received (e.g., type(s) of medications prescribed, diagnostic tests done, purpose(s) of encounters, dietary or exercise instructions, referrals made, etc.). In medical emergencies, consumers may be unable to provide information important to beginning appropriate treatment in a timely fashion (e.g., blood type, next of kin, current family doctor, chronic conditions, allergies, current medications, treatment to date).

The encounter card could provide an important vehicle for consumers to communicate more efficiently and effectively with health service providers about their health problems and needs. It also would allow more rapid, appropriate response by health providers to patients' needs in a medical emergency when time is an important factor. Further, consumers, who will have knowledge of the information contained on their personal card, will have a greater awareness of the types of health-care interventions received and their current medications. Since compliance with health-care advice is sometimes hampered by a patient's lack of understanding, patient compliance may also be enhanced.

Parents also have difficulty accurately recalling the health-care histories of their children, their medications, dates/types of immunizations. The ready availability of such information on their children's cards will be of assistance to them.

It was anticipated that the benefits to consumers of an encounter card would be greatest for those who have chronic medical conditions, are taking several medications, require care from several providers or agencies and/or develop emergency health-care problems.

Health-care providers and agencies. The development of an encounter card for consumers also has several potential benefits for providers. Such a health encounter card could provide information about the patient in a medical emergency, facilitate history taking and communication with patients, and generally provide a quick reference to health conditions, health services provided and ordered for a patient as well as current medications. It was expected to improve communication within and among provider groups and assist in the management of complicated conditions that involve many providers. As well, the information used to capture encounters could provide a convenient summary of patient care activities, referral sources and dispositions of those referrals for each provider/agency.

The encounter card might provide an efficient way for physicians to capture prescription renewals for their records and assist in avoiding prescription of medications and medical interventions that have caused problems for the patient previously. Information on the card could assist in avoiding duplication of service by providers and assist in identification of patient compliance problems. The health encounter card could facilitate the development of computerized office/agency-based health-care records. This might also allow the development of other types of memory aids for the provider (e.g., immunization update reminder, drug interaction warning system, etc.) within the provider's practice. Finally, the standard record of care given could support efficient peer review of activities within a group of health-care providers.

Ministry of Health. Because the encounter record is completed at the time of the encounter (or shortly thereafter) more timely information should be available to the Ministry of Health than the current reporting systems allow. Further, assuming that the encounter card is eventually linked to, or is a subset of, the individual patient record of physicians and other health-care providers, improvement in the quality of information regarding the type(s) of health-care problems seen should also occur which could facilitate better planning for health-care needs. The encounter record also will identify which services were rendered, authorized or ordered for which types of conditions. This linkage is difficult to determine in the current system, even with the addition of a unique health service number. Since the system will identify the date a consultation request or referral decision was made as well as when the request/referral was actually carried out for the patient, the encounter record has the potential to identify bottlenecks in the health-care delivery system. Again, this should enhance the planning capabilities of the Ministry of Health and District Health Councils.

The Ministry of Health recently published *Mandatory Health Programs and Service Standards for Public Health Units.*[8] As part of these guidelines Public Health Units are required to assess and keep records of the immunization status of all children at school entry and annually thereafter to ensure that they are immunized (or have been exempted from immunization). They are also required to assess annually the immunization status of children in licensed child-care programs.

The availability of computer readable personal health cards for all children would facilitate the Public Health Units' task. The Pharmaceutical Inquiry of Ontario strongly recommended that a drug utilization review capability become part of the Ontario health data collect systems.[9] Information is not presently available about ongoing patterns of the prescription and utilization of drugs for various age groups, disease categories and geographic areas of the province. Information generated could assist physicians and pharmacists in their evaluation of treatment patterns, help establish dynamic standards of care on a drug-by-drug basis while helping to reduce the number of prescription drugs diverted to illegal street drug traffic. The health encounter card could support drug utilization review because it provides information on all drugs prescribed concurrently, and the diagnosis leading to the prescription. Obviously safeguards would need to be in place to assure patient confidentiality and possibly anonymity in the use of data.

Professional bodies. Professional bodies have several responsibilities that may benefit from the types of information generated from encounter cards: monitoring of adherence to standards of care by the members (quality assurance); development of new standards or guidelines for care; and provision of timely continuing education to members.

Currently, these functions are often hampered because easily retrieved, uniform, patient-based information is not available about health-care activities of providers and the patterns of care sought out by consumers. Regulatory bodies often lack information about the types of health-care problems that their members are asked to address in a given type of setting. They have little data about the variability across providers in their management of specific health-care problems. Review of paper records of care for quality assurance purposes is costly, labour intensive and often unsatisfactory, as the information and its location in the record are not standardized.

Health Care Researchers. The encounter data collected with the card provide both an integrated record of care at the patient level and higher quality information (because they are used for communication purposes as well as administrative purposes). This permits more and higher quality health-care research. It could allow researchers to generate new knowledge important to understanding and improving the health of the population and health care in Ontario. Health-care researchers are often interested in describing patterns of care and factors that appear to influence those patterns and in examining the relative effectiveness or efficiency of various health-care services and delivery systems. They are also interested in how health-care information or technology disseminates, as well as the factors that hamper or aid that dissemination. Such activities are hampered by unreliability of recorded diagnoses. The health encounter card could support study of referral and communication patterns among providers and between provider and consumer. Studies of the natural history of diseases and the effects of different courses of care could also be done. Such information is needed by both the health professions and government to develop new initiatives and policies.

Decision rules must be developed to ensure that data are available at suitable levels of aggregation for use in research and that unique patient and provider identifiers are removed or altered to protect the anonymity of both consumers and providers/agencies.

PROJECT DEVELOPMENT AND IMPLEMENTATION

The pilot project was designed to be a six-month field test of the health encounter card system. An advisory committee was struck by the Ministry of Health to oversee project development. It included representatives from key constituencies including district health councils, hospitals, health professions, and the Ministry of Health. This group provided the expertise (or access to the expertise) necessary to design the pilot, to select the pilot situation, to develop a community awareness program, to direct the pilot and to evaluate its effectiveness. Two working groups were organized, overseen by the Advisory Committee. One group focused on site selection and the approach to the local community. The other worked through the operational plans for the project: studying data elements to be included on the card and part of the encounter record system, and how they would be coded; as well as examining policies and procedures to ensure confidentiality of health information and to proscribe access to such information. Once basic decisions had been made about these matters (described in more detail below) and a site was chosen, a local advisory group was formed to review the plans and continue to modify them to fit local circumstances. For example, final decisions regarding the scope of providers to be included were negotiated with the site chosen. As well, all operational details were discussed with the local community and its expertise was used.

Pilot Site Selection

The first working group was charged with the task of recommending possible sites for the pilot project. Desirable characteristics of a potential location were seen as: an area with a population-base of under 50,000 with a fairly stable year-round population; a range of services locally available — including hospital, home care, pharmacy; and both primary and some secondary level health services. The site should not be near a large centre so that many people would likely work and seek health-care services outside the immediate area. Finally, the local community chosen must be interested and willing to serve as a pilot site. This led to the selection of Fort Frances and Emo; two adjacent communities and their surrounding area in northern Ontario which share many of their health-care services but are geographically fairly isolated from other larger centres.

Description of the Basic Operational Concepts of the Project

Defining an encounter. One of the early tasks in developing the project was to define the term "health-care encounter." An encounter was defined as an interaction between a patient and a provider for the delivery of a health service at a given time and place. It included an examination and treatment by a physician or other health professional; laboratory and other diagnostic tests; filling of a prescription; home-care visit; admission to hospital; and any other contacts aimed at maintaining, restoring or improving the health state of the individual.

Defining the Elements of an Encounter. Information about service encounters was seen as crucial to planning, funding and evaluating the health-care system. In examining options for the encounter system, the elements and coding schemes of other encounter-based systems were reviewed.[10] A meeting was organized with members of the academic community in Ontario who were interested in health services research and planning in order to obtain their input.[11] Another working group was identified to work through the details of the encounter record, the patient encounter card and its implementation in a pilot study. This working group included representatives from major health professional groups (medicine, nursing and pharmacy), hospitals, district health councils charged with health planning for their regions and MOH officials. Here issues were discussed regarding the elements necessary for inclusion (and their coding schemes), and how the system could be implemented in the field. Safeguards were developed to ensure confidentiality of information, and policies and procedures to restrict access to some types of information.

The basic elements describing a service encounter were defined to include information about the (a) patient and provider which could be gained directly from the patient and provider cards; (b) the time and date of the encounter, the facility or place of encounter, and the funding program that would be available from the local computer; and (c) the information about the encounter that would be completed at the time of the encounter. Basic elements included the source of referral, the services or procedures provided, the diagnoses (up to three) responsible for the visit, medications received (if any), referrals made and provider comments (if any). (See Table 4:1.)

Table 4:1. *Elements of Service Encounter Data*

Date/Time of Encounter Hospital/Agency Place of Visit Postal Code of Site Program Funding	To be supplied by local work station

Patient Information
  Sex
  Health Number+
  Birthdate/Age
	To be obtained from
	patient encounter card

Patient Type°	

Authorizing Provider
  ID Number
  Specialty
  Service Provider
	To be supplied by
	provider card

Source of Referral Services/Procedures Provided and Quantity (where applicable)	
Diagnosis or Symptoms* Medications* Referral Options* Provider Comments	To be completed at time of encounter

°Important for hospital use only
*Field may be slightly changed or omitted, depending on type of provider.
+Patient confidentiality is protected by transforming the health number to another unique number within the pilot encounter database.

Source: Authors' compilation.

Types of Information to be Included on the Health Encounter Card

The health encounter card was designed to contain a comprehensive personal health-care record. It includes basic biographic information, information useful in medical emergencies — including vital medical history — and personal and private health information; as well as history of service encounters, particularly recent or very important ones. (See Table 4:2.)

Table 4:2. *Data Elements to be Included on The Encounter Card: A Personal, Portable Health Record*

Biographic Data

Health Number	Birthdate
Name	Sex
Address	Official language used
Language usually spoken	

Emergency Contact Information

Primary physician, name and phone number
Emergency contact name and phone numbers
Blood type

Vital Medical History

Drug sensitivities and other allergies
Immunization record

Personal and Private Information

Medical/health problems
Chronic conditions
Significant test results
Family history
Provider notes

Service Encounter History

Current medications (30)
Expired medications
Medical service encounters (12)
Hospital service encounters (in hospital) (3)
Radiology encounters (4)
Laboratory encounters (7)
Allied health-care encounters (8)

() Number given in brackets is the maximum number the encounter card will hold in each category. Encounters will be stored on the MOH central database.

Source: Authors' compilation.

It is much more than simply a collection of service encounter data. The health encounter card, a portable health record, is a tool in the hands of the patient and provider to support the delivery of health care. It has the potential to consolidate significant health details that exist today in the files of multiple providers and to share information that otherwise would not be available among authorized providers.

Only the service encounters recorded on the card support the creation of a comprehensive service delivery database to assist the MOH and other health-care planners in effective planning and evaluation of the health-care system. Even here, there may not be one-to-one mapping of service encounter details on the card to that collected for planning. Only a portion of the information found on the card which relates to encounters is contributed to the central database with the patient's permission. Some information found in the central database will be truncated on the card. Certain planning-specific data are recorded only in the project service encounter (e.g., MOH program that provides funding). In some cases service encounters on the card are aggregates or summaries of the encounters. For example, during the pilot, individual physiotherapy service encounters will be captured in the MOH database for pilot evaluation purposes. The encounter card, however, will contain a single encounter record that identifies the provider, the date treatment began, the last visit date, the service provided at that time and optionally, a provider note. Detailed listing of laboratory tests performed on the encounter card is also impractical. The OHIP *Schedule of Benefits* provides a discrete code for each test. Physicians may order a battery of tests (e.g., complete blood counts, cardiac enzymes, etc.). To avoid problems created by limited storage space on the card and to make the description of laboratory tests more "patient friendly," simplified coding terms such as "Complete Blood Counts" (used to describe haemoglobin, haematocrit, white blood count, red blood count and platelets) were substituted on the health encounter card record of laboratory tests provided although the MOH database collects the actual laboratory tests performed using OHIP codes.

The encounter card can also serve as a data access key to information not directly contained on the card. Results of laboratory and other diagnostic tests will not be routinely included on the card because the results of such tests are usually not immediately available at the time that patients present their cards to obtain the service. Even without any results actually being stored on the card, it can provide a secure means to share information among authorized providers by identifying when and where the tests were done, with the patient remaining in control of the process. The patient and physician may later decide to store significant normal or abnormal results, that would be helpful for themselves or other authorized practitioners whom the patient is to visit subsequently, in the significant test results section of the card.

Policies and Procedures for Ensuring Confidentially of Information During Implementation

To access a patient's health encounter card, a valid health provider card must be placed in the card reader which is attached to a computer work station at the provider's work site. Participating health-care providers are registered and receive provider access cards and personal identification numbers (PINs) that permit them to read and update (write to) the patient card. Health-care providers will only have access to the information that they need to ensure the proper care of the patient. Which fields of the card are open to a given provider depends on his/her discipline as encrypted on the provider card, as well as in an access rights table which is secured in the provider work station. Security and confidentiality of patient cards are maintained because these cards can only be read or modified at a work station provided by the project, in conjunction with a provider card that has a valid PIN. A special work station is also planned in a secure location for registered pilot project patients to view the information on their cards after identifying themselves as the valid card holder. (Other pilots have demonstrated that patients are very interested in the information contained on their cards.)[12]

Patients may choose not to have an encounter recorded on their health-care encounter card or transmitted to the project's central database. The central database will not record the patient's name. The patient's health number will be recorded as a transformed number. Patients may receive services without their card being present. Such encounters would be stored on the provider work station for later updating of the card, for example, when the patient next returns to visit the provider.

The pilot will only collect medication data if the patient has presented his/her card to the pharmacist; card presentation represents patient consent to record and collect such data. Prescriptions recorded by the pharmacist in the pilot will contain a prescribing physician identified to assist in linkage of prescriptions to medical service encounters. Although both medications covered and not covered by the Ontario Drug Benefit Plan will appear on the card, the pilot database will only collect encounter data for Ontario Drug Benefit Plan prescriptions. This is another example of the somewhat different information collected by the card and the MOH data systems.

Any printout made in a participating physician's office of encounters that have occurred since the last visit (visits to pharmacy, lab, by home care, etc.) will be treated as part of the patient's usual medical record. This printout function is available to physicians who opt not to review card data directly on their work stations. As well, the physician may opt to print out a copy of the encounter for the patient's paper medical record. On request, a paper copy would also be available to the patient.

Enrolment of Consumers

Attention also focused on how to best communicate to consumers the operational concepts and rationale for the project. Decisions had to be made regarding how the descriptive material should be presented, the contents of the enrolment form, the consent required for participation and the amount of historical health information to be directly obtained from each participating consumer. Legal consultation was required to formulate the consent procedures. Each potential enrolee received an enrolment kit that contained a brochure describing the project and a security and privacy fact sheet, along with a letter from the primary care provider about the project. The application form requested the consumer's name, address, telephone number, health card number, name style preference; the name and location of their primary physician; and name and telephone numbers of a person to contact in case of emergency. The decision was taken that historical health information included on cards would be abstracted from primary care physicians' records and checked by the physicians for accuracy. Thus, such information was not obtained directly from consumers.

A series of information sessions were also publicized and held in each community to allow the public to ask any specific questions that they had about the project and their potential role. Enrolment of participants proceeded before implementation so that consumers could be issued cards. Implementation began on 29 June 1992.

Enrolment of Providers

Health-care providers included in the pilot project area were approached about their willingness to participate. A provider enrolment form was also required to ensure that each provider understood the nature of the project, the expectations of the project, its rationale and basic operating concepts. Some local providers also served on the community advisory committee and helped work through specific implementation issues.

Other Implementation Issues

The complex nature of the encounter card pilot spawned a plethora of implementation issues. Although most of these issues had been anticipated in advance, the time needed to address them and find acceptable solutions was still significant. Two of such issues are described below.

Decisions had to be taken regarding how existing coding schemes (Schedule of Benefits used by physicians; the Hospital Medical Records Institute (HMRI) coding system and workload measurement systems employed in hospitals), could be linked and adapted to minimize duplication of effort in recording. Although the International Classification of Primary Care [13] was the initial prototype shown to physicians for diagnostic codes, a three digit level coding of the ICD-9 [14] was adopted to avoid the need to train physicians and health records staff in hospitals who were already familiar with ICD-9. The ICD-9 also maps very closely to the diagnostic codes used by the Ontario Health Insurance Plan.[15] The medical records department of the hospital provides regular reporting to HMRI, using the ICD-9 codes for diagnoses and the codes contained in the Canadian Classification of Diagnostic, Therapeutic and Surgical Procedures (CCP) [16] for therapeutic and surgical procedures. However, OHIP *Schedule of Benefits*[17] codes are used to code diagnostic imaging techniques. Hospital laboratory staff are familiar with OHIP *Schedule of Benefits* codes for laboratory services and the medical laboratory in the community clinic uses OHIP codes. A hybrid system of coding was eventually adopted. ICD-9 is used to code diagnoses; CCP is used for procedures and OHIP *Schedule of Benefits* codes are used for the remainder of service descriptors. However, the descriptions of some OHIP codes were simplified to make them more patient friendly and a few new codes had to be added to describe services not covered in the OHIP *Schedule of Benefits*.

Another implementation issue was the technical problems involved in interfacing existing computer hardware and software in community pharmacies with project software. The retail pharmacists, who all use computers as an integral part of their business, required a fully integrated solution that would permit them to read and update a patient encounter card with minimal interruption to their normal methods for recording of a prescription. This sometimes requires the upgrading of existing hardware and software to provide good performance. Pharmacists have also raised concerns about prompting customers for their health encounter cards for fear of embarrassing a customer who does not want to use the card for the encounter.

Scope of Pilot Project

Not all of the potential benefits of health encounter cards could be explored in this project because it is limited both in the size of the population studied and the relatively brief (six-month) length of time the project is to be in the field. The inclusion of a broad cross-section of people from the local community and representation from diverse health-care provider groups and agencies allow the project to assess how well this health-care application is accepted by both consumers and by different types of health-care providers.

Approximately 2,300 residents of the Emo and Fort Frances area volunteered to be enroled and received health encounter cards. This represents about one in nine people in this region. While the majority of patients reside in Emo and Fort Frances, a significant number are from surrounding towns such as Mine River, Devlin and Nestor Falls. Volunteers also include native Canadians from local reserves.

In Emo, three pharmacists and two physicians who work at the medical centre and the nurses from Northwestern Home Care agreed to participate. A portable computer is used by home care nurses while the other providers have regular work stations on site. In Fort Frances, three community pharmacies, Northwestern Home Care, Northwestern Health Unit, an optometrist and 13 physicians associated with the Fort Frances Clinic are involved in the project. The local hospital, La Verendrye General Hospital, also agreed to participate. Again, nurses associated with home care use a portable computer. Public health nurses also use portable computers to update immunization records on encounter cards when they visit schools for an immunization clinic. Eight work stations are available at La Venerdrye General Hospital. Admissions and discharges are recorded as well as encounters in the emergency room, physician encounters, diagnostic imaging, laboratory and pharmacy encounters and selected encounters with other health professionals in the outpatient department. Family and Children's Services, the local child welfare agency, is participating indirectly be registering some of the foster children in their care to carry health encounter cards.

Evaluation Plans and Procedures

The evaluation design addressed three areas of central concern in this pilot project:

- concerns about acceptability and compliance by patients and providers;
- issues regarding the process of using the service encounter cards (confidentiality, communication patterns, empowerment); and

- benefits realized through use of the service encounter cards (use in medical emergencies and drug management).

Two data collection periods have been defined: one during the pilot, two months after initial implementation, and one at the conclusion of the project. Three types of data will be collected at the two-month point:

- Telephone interviews will be conducted with drop-outs from the pilot project, both patients and providers. It is reasonable to expect that various patients and providers may discontinue participation after initial willingness. A telephone interview with each of these individuals will document the reason for opting out. Telephone interviews will be both more complete and more likely to return the information than would be a written questionnaire.

- Focus groups will be held with providers to supply process improvement information. The purpose of these groups is to identify ongoing problems and to develop potential solutions. Both positive aspects of the system (avoidance of dangerous drug interactions, increased access to other health-care encounters or problems) as well as negative aspects (card failure, information delays, concerns about confidentiality) will be elicited during these group discussions.

- Additional mid-project information will be gathered through focus groups with a selected cross-section of the patients involved in the project. This cross-section will be chosen across levels and types of participants and will focus on identifying problems and solutions to issues of confidentiality, usability, interaction with providers and increased participant empowerment.

At the pilot conclusion, data collection will again be of three types:

- A written questionnaire will be administered to a selection of participating consumers and all providers at the conclusion of the six-month pilot. These questionnaires will be created to provide an opportunity for consumers and providers to comment on all the key evaluation areas of importance in this pilot. A stratified random sample of 1,000 consumers will be drawn to ensure representation of target patient groups. All providers will be requested to complete and return a second questionnaire. The creation and fine tuning of the questions included in each questionnaire, one for consumers and the second for providers, will be carefully based on input and feedback obtained throughout the project from all involved sources.

- Interviews will be organized with each of the 35 providers at the conclusion of the pilot. This will ensure detailed responses to important topics and to difficult topics, those, therefore unlikely to receive full response in the questionnaire (for example, an estimation and detail on the number of times a provider changed a drug prescription based on the personal health record available).

- Focus groups involving the providers will also be held at the conclusion of the pilot. These group sessions will have the purpose of cross-professional and cross-provider discussion and communication about pilot project outcomes including changes in interactions between themselves and patients, perceived empowerment of patients, changes in communication among providers, improved management of medical emergencies due to improved access to vital information, and improved drug management. These focus groups will also identify remaining problems with acceptance and compliance, security and confidentiality.

In addition to this data collection focused on providers and consumers, the pilot project will also collect process evaluation information about the technical operations and reliability of this system. Process evaluation plans include monitoring the technical operations and reliability of the system (e.g., number of card malfunctions, number of full cards, reader malfunction, etc.). Freedom of information regulations will not allow an assessment of how often encounters occur that are not captured on the health encounter card. Providers will be encouraged to use a diary function to describe both positive aspects of the system (e.g., avoid potential drug interaction, provide useful information about other encounters or problems) and negative aspects (e.g., card failure, delays).

CONCLUSIONS

The time frame for the pilot test (six months) will place significant bounds on how many of the potential benefits of a health encounter card system can be assessed. The project should provide an adequate test of the feasibility of the collection of health encounter data and the acceptance, reliability and security of the health encounter card technology. Feedback to the MOH, providers and others with respect to the impact of the technology on the business of the various stakeholders should be gleaned. Both in the planning phase and during implementation, the encounter card project has already assisted in the analysis of issues related to data standards, data usage and operational concerns related to implementing an encounter-based information system across different providers and settings. It will test whether we can develop for the first time, on a timely basis, health service profiles by individuals, providers, geographic location, diagnosis, type of care, etc., from an encounter database.

Notes

The authors wish to thank Dan McKenna for his comments and suggestions.

[1]See M.E. Hayken and R.B.J. Warner, *Smart Card Technology: New Methods for Computer Access Control*, NIST Special Publication 500-157 (Garthersburg, MD: National Institute of Standards and Technology, 1988).

[2]P. Bannister, "Computer Readable Personal Health Cards: Development in Other Countries," Appendix H in Section 1B, Conference Proceedings: Symposium on Personal Health Cards, 2 and 3 May 1990 (Winnipeg: Manitoba Health Communications Branch).

[3]See H.J. Segal and T.R. Einerson, "An Evaluation of the Use of Smart Cards by Community Pharmacists," unpublished document submitted to Greenshields Prepaid Services, Inc., Ontario Pharmacists' Association and Veterans Affairs Canada.

[4]For the project at Laval, see J.P. Fortin, C. Boudreau, G. Lavoie, J. Berube, A. Gamache and M.P. Papillion, *The Quebec Patient Smart Card (PSC) Project: Managing an Innovating Technology*, fourth Global Congress on Patient Cards, May 1992, Berlin, Germany. A. Wyszkowski, "Health Care Applications of Card Technology in Canada," Appendix G, Conference Proceedings: Symposium on Personal Health Cards, 2 and 3 May 1990 (Winnipeg: Manitoba Health Communications Branch) reviews the information from North Vancouver.

[5]Ontario Health Review Panel, *Toward a Shared Direction for Health in Ontario*, J. Evans, Chairman (Toronto: Ministry of Health, 1987); *Health Promotion Matters in Ontario*, S. Podworski, Chairman (Toronto: Ontario Ministry of Health, 1987); and Panel on Health Goals for Ontario, *Health for All Ontario*, R. Spasoff, Chairman (Toronto: Ministry of Health, 1987).

[6]See Ontario, Ministry of Health, Information and Systems Division, *Information and Technology Strategic Plan* (Toronto: Ministry of Health, 1989).

[7]Ontario, Ministry of Health, Information Systems Division, *Corporate Service Encounter Data Requirements: Conceptual and Logical Data Models*; *Implementation Strategy* (Toronto: Ministry of Health, 1990).

[8]Ontario Ministry of Health, *Mandatory Health Programs and Service Guidelines* (Toronto: Ministry of Health, 1989).

[9]Pharmaceutical Inquiry of Ontario, *Final Report*, F. Lowy, Chairman (Toronto: Ministry of Health, 1990).

[10]See H. Lambert and H. Woods (eds.), *International Classification of Primary care* (New York: Oxford University Press, 1987); and J. Read and T. Benson, "Comprehensive Coding," *British Journal of Health Care Computing* 3(2): 22-25.

[11]See J. Dorland, "Report on the Proceedings of a Workshop on Data for Health Care Planning, Policy, Development and Applied Research" (Kingston: Department of Community Health and Epidemiology, Queen's University, 1990).

[12]M.S. Hall and R.J. Hopkins, "Interim Evaluation Exeter Care Card Trial: Exeter Care Card Project" (Exeter: University of Exeter Postgraduate Medical School, 1990).

[13]Lambert and Woods, *International Classification of Primary Care.*

[14]World Health Organization, *International Classification of Disease: Manual of the International Classification of Diseases, Injuries and Causes of Death*, rev. (Geneva: World Health Organization, 1977).

[15]Ontario, Ministry of Health, *Diagnostic Codes Listed Alphabetically and Numerically* (Toronto: Ministry of Health, 1987).

[16]Statistics Canada, Health Division, Nosology Reference Centre, *Canadian Classification of Diagnostic, Therapeutic and Surgical Procedures* (Ottawa: Minister of Supply and Services, 1986).

[17]Ontario, Ministry of Health, *OHIP Schedule of Benefits: Physicians' Services* (Toronto: Ministry of Health, 1989).

5

The Reform of the Quebec Health-Care System: Potential for Innovation?

Raynald Pineault

When I was asked almost a year ago to give this paper on health-care reform in Quebec, I did not realize what the task would be because nobody knew at that time what the reform would look like in its final version.

As you know, we have become used to reforms in Quebec especially in the health-care sector, and we are never sure if they bring about real changes and innovations or only, in Allport's terms, dynamics without change.

The title of this paper is: "The Reform of the Quebec Health-Care system: Potential for Innovation?" Note the question mark at the end. Note also the term "potential for innovation" because the major elements of the reform do not necessarily refer to innovative concepts, but when looked at in the processes that have led to their adoption, and in their relationship with contextual factors that I will discuss later they constitute innovation and they have certainly created a potential for innovation.

The framework I suggest for analyzing health-care reform is simple. As shown in Chart 5:1 the starting point is the problems identified for justifying a reform, and more specifically, some elements of the reform, since I have selected five elements of the reform that I judged to be the most important or central. I will present these elements later on. The framework thus presents five elements of the reform that were proposed in response to the problems identified. Those measure should bring about changes or results as shown in the framework under "expected impact" and solve the problems as shown by the feedback dotted line. Finally, the analysis of the reform cannot be done in a closed system perspective without looking at its environment, that is at conditions, internal and external to the health system, that can make the reform a success or a failure.

Following this framework, what I have to say goes as follows. First, in order to understand the context in which current reform is taking place, I will present a brief overview of the historical evolution of the Quebec health-care system in the last two decades, that is following the Castonguay Commission in the early 1970s. Second, I will describe five major elements of the current reform in relation to the problems they intend to solve. Third, for each of these elements, I will discuss the challenges associated with the implementation of reform, both in terms of conditions of failure and of success. Finally, I will analyze some general contextual factors that may also facilitate or jeopardize the implementation of the reform.

Chart 5:1. *Framework for the Analysis of the Quebec Health-Care Reform*

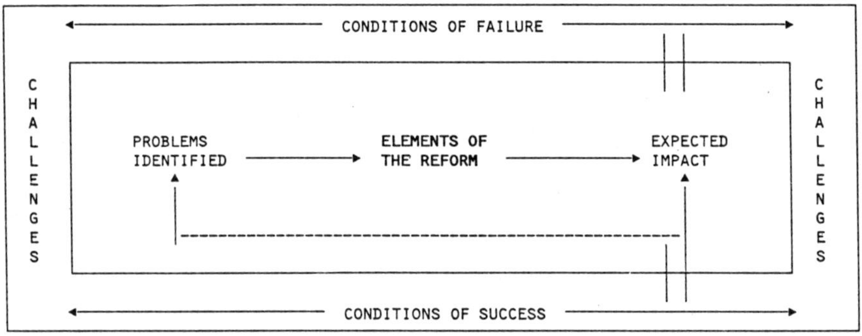

Source: Author's compilation.

HISTORICAL BACKGROUND OF THE REFORM

Let us begin with an historical overview of the evolution of the Quebec health-care system in the last two decades.[1]

In Quebec, a reform of the health system was carried out in the early 1970s following the recommendations of the Commission of Inquiry of Health and Social Services, also known as the Castonguay-Nepveu Commission.[2]

The Castonguay-Nepveu Report led in particular to the adhesion of Quebec to the Canadian national health insurance scheme. The plan also brought in legislated changes affecting the professions, the organization of health-care delivery, and the administration of health services. A few health-care organizations were eliminated (public health units); some had their role and functions redefined (the Department of Social Affairs and the professional corporations), while many others were created. Among these, a network of organizations known as CLSCs (local community health services centres), offering primary health and social services, was created. Public Health and preventive services were delegated to departments of Community Health (DSC) located in 32 hospitals; the province was subdivided into 12 regions under the jurisdiction of regional councils (CRSSS) but their responsibilities were limited.

In 1985, as a result of the economic slowdown and in response to the major strain exerted by health-care expenditures on the public funds, the Quebec government authorized a second commission of inquiry chaired by Jean Rochon to evaluate the functioning and financing of the health and social services systems.[3] This was the first step in a process that would lead to a second reform. The major findings of the Rochon Commission were: (a) overall good performance of our health-care system in terms of health indicators and control of health-care costs; (b) good quality of care; (c) high satisfaction of the population; as well as (d) difficulty of adjust to changing needs of the population; (e) not enough decentalization; and (f) not enough citizen participation since the system has become the hostage of the countless interest groups.

In its report, tabled at the end of 1987, the Rochon Commission provided a wide-ranging review of the Quebec health system and recommended a major reform. The Rochon Commission's assessment was based on both a very detailed analysis of the data available and on extensive consultations with the public and groups representing the principal actors in the system.

This assessment contained mixed findings. On the one hand, in general the Quebec health-care system was judged as healthy in terms of its evolution as compared to other health-care systems. On the other hand, several deficiencies were identified. Specifically, the following points emerged:

- health-care expenditures are relatively high in Quebec, representing 9 percent of the GNP (greater than the Canadian average, greater than the majority of OECD countries, but much less than the United States);

- the growth of these expenditures has been kept under control since the introduction of the public health insurance system;

- the state covers a major portion of health-care expenditures (approximately 80 percent). However, since 1978 there is evidence of a slow but steady withdrawal of the government of Quebec in the financing of health care;

- the overall indicators of health in the Quebec population have progressed more quickly than in the majority of OECD countries;

- as a whole, the performance of the Quebec health-care system is very good as compared to that of the OECD countries;

- regional accessibility of health services has improved despite persistent considerable interregional discrepancies for specialized services;

- the public network of CLSCs covers the entire province (158 are currently in operation). This alternative model of integrated health care and social services introduces competition in a mixed public-private system and is a positive factor for innovation;

- the overall level of resources available per capita (physicians, hospitals, technologies) is high;

- the technical quality of the medical care is high and meets North American standards for modern medicine;

- public satisfaction with the health system in general is higher than that observed in other countries;

- public satisfaction with services provided by physicians is high; and

- professionals, particularly physicians, are mostly satisfied with the Quebec health insurance system, although they are concerned about the relative stagnation of their income levels.

Given that positive assessment of our health-care system by the Commission, why then recommend a vast reform?

First, there is what I would call a change bias in any social and political process. Once initiated, the process must bring about changes, and the longer it lasts, the more important the changes must be. Let me illustrate that by an anecdote. Before the Commission made public its final report, the Commissioners organized a two-day meeting with consultants who had not been directly involved in the Commission's work. I was one of them, the least experienced I must say, along with people of great reputation and expertise, such as John Hasting, Sid Lee, Jacques Brunet, and a few others. We endorsed the overall assessment of the Commission but we feel that minor changes could be made to improve our system at the margins. The president of the Commission reacted to that view by arguing that the government had invested too much in the Commission to be simply told that overall our system was doing well and that changes should be introduced slowly, progressively and just at the margins.

Of course, changes to be recommended must be based on identified problems. Although the Rochon Commission considered that the positive elements in the system had to be protected, its observations did not end there. It was troubled by the increasing difficulty the system was experiencing to adjust to the changing needs of the population, to motivate its personnel, to redistribute the powers and functions of the various bodies to better serve the public, to foster participation of citizens in decision making, to decentralize its management, and to reconsider its financing to improve the delivery of services and the efficiency of the system.

It was as if the system had become the hostage or the prisoner of the countless interest groups concerned with health care: groups of producers, groups of institutions, groups of community-based activists, unions, and so forth. It often seemed as if only the law of survival of the fittest applied and that the democratic arbitration mechanisms were no longer sufficient. It was as if the person to be helped, the population to be served, the needs to be met, the problems to be solved, in short the common good had been lost to the specific interests of these various groups.

In agreement with this analysis, the Commission recommended that the system be more centred on the individuals rather than on the providers. In particular, it recommended that regional councils be replaced by regional bodies that would be granted the power of direct taxation and whose members would be elected by universal ballot. In other words, the Commission opted for a true political decentralization rather than only an administrative one.

The politicians, who were expecting recommendations on the day-to-day problems of the system did not receive the report of the Commission with overwhelming enthusiasm. Indeed, the public, the popular press and elected officials were very sensitive to some system operational dysfunctions which they felt did not receive enough direct attention from the Commission. These included: insufficient availability of long-term care; local problems of waiting time for elective admission to acute-care hospitals, caused in large part by the fact that occupancy rates are maintained at a too-high level because of the inability to discharge patients to long-term care; bottlenecks in some hospitals' emergency rooms, also caused in part by the same problem and in part by the tendency of the population and of physicians to use hospitals' emergency rooms for problems that would be more suitably handled in other ambulatory settings. Similarly, the medical profession and the influential interest groups, who were expecting recommendations of increased financing, also gave the report a chilly reception.

The minister of health at the time, Therese Lavoie-Roux, promised to make concrete proposals for reform before the end of her mandate. In April 1989, the minister issued a document entitled "Orientations"; it suggested that the health system be reorganized around outcome objectives and that it should rely on an increased mobilization of the various participants and the population. This plan, which called for strong decentralization, was put on the shelves because of provincial elections. In 1990, a new minister of health, Marc-Yvan Côté, initiated the reform process with the publication of a White Paper, "A Reform Focusing on the Citizen," and pledged to implement reform that would solve effectively the genuine problems. According to the minister, the issues included re-establishing the individual at the centre of the system, limiting the power of professionals and institutions, and redirecting the system in relation to outcome objectives.

As some elements will be detailed later on, the proposed reform of December 1990 contained the following elements: establishing regional boards with a board of directors on which the majority of the members were to be citizens and thus responsible for allocation of resources and planning of services in each territory; resorting to the user fee to halt the inappropriate use of hospital emergency rooms, introducing the concept of services as taxable income; decentralizing regionally the budgets for remuneration of physicians to promote better geographic distribution of manpower; establishing a certification procedure for physicians practising in private offices; requiring patients' signatures on physicians' fee statements; creating a system to hear user complaints; eliminating, to a large extent, the medical-administrative structure in institutions; restructuring the nursing home and rehabilitation sector; creating common boards for institutions with fewer than 50 beds in a single region; and formally recognizing the role of community organizations.

The physicians reacted strongly to this plan (public relations campaign, work stoppages, and so on). They objected on the grounds that it interfered in the doctor-patient relationship, decreased their decision-making role in institutions, excluded them from the regional boards, and resorted to coercion to promote better distribution of physicians throughout the province. In short, for them the reform represented an attempt to subjugate the medical profession to technocratic authority. Illustrative of this was the disposition that placed the

Medical Board under the authority of the Executive Director rather than the Board of Directors.

The other actors reacted more favourably on the overall project, but tended to secure their own position by proposing various amendments, which contributed considerably to the lengthening of the final Bill that was adopted, passing from 494 articles in the initial version to 622 in the final one. Every group agreed with the proposed reform as long as its position was maintained and protected. The Quebec Hospital Association (AHQ) appreciated the strengthening of the authority of administrators over physicians and the resorting to alternative sources of financing. Nevertheless, it criticized the reform for compartmentalizing the mission of the institutions, with the hospitals to play only a curative role and for the bureaucratization that the regional boards might entail. The Federation of CLSCs saw the reform as a shift in the health system towards prevention objectives and greater recognition of their role. But it was against both the user fee and the service tax. The Quebec Association of Nursing Homes (ACAQ) (including institutions in the nursing home and rehabilitation sectors) was also very positive towards the reform since it favoured greater complementary interventions in this sector. The Confederation of Regional Councils (the future regional boards) supported the principle of giving citizens a greater part in the system, but stressed the risk of increased bureaucratization and centralization as if it was an inevitable process over which they had no control. The Association of Executive Directors in the health-care network supported the measures intended to reduce the power of physicians, but were apprehensive about losing administrative autonomy.

Confronted with the organized resistance of the physicians, and lacking the clear support of many other groups, the state agreed to negotiate the reform. Obviously, the political context may well have played an important role as the government was then confronted with other more important issues, at least from the premier's point of view, namely the constitutional crisis and the relationships with the First Nations. Any confrontation with the medical profession was to be avoided, at any price. The negotiating process lasted several months and led to adoption of Bill 120 on 28 August 1991. This reform relies on regionalization, but manages to avoid coercing the medical profession. In fact, through the creation of the regional boards, it solidly establishes the principle of a regional organization of services subject to ministerial approval. The legislation rejects both the user fee and the principle of the service tax, thus effectively postponing the debate on the health-system financing. It limits the autonomy of institutions and forces them to respect whatever is approved at the regional level or suffer administrative sanctions.

The physicians were able to get the state to bend on several points: no regionalization of a closed budget for their remuneration; postponement of

decisions concerning their geographic distribution until April 1993; postponement of certification in private offices; preservation of the medical-administrative structures in institutions and a guarantee of their representation on the
different decision-making bodies. In short, to a large extent, the physicians
were able to maintain their pre-reform position, but the minister maintained
the sword of Damocles over their head since all those dispositions, while not
enforced, were kept in the Bill. If the physicians do not meet the 1993 deadline,
the minister has the right to strike again and this time irrevocably.

MAIN ELEMENTS OF THE REFORM AND PROBLEMS IT AIMED TO SOLVE

After this brief historical overview of the current reform of health-care in
Quebec, rather than trying to identify and analyze the overall potential of the
reform for generating innovations, I decided to be more specific and focus on
five elements of the reform that seem to me more original and more capable
of generating innovations. I will first present each of these elements and the
problems it aims to solve. Then following the framework presented earlier, I
will try to assess the potential of the elements of the reforms for generating
innovations in the system. Finally the role of contextual factors associated with
the success or failure of their implementation will be discussed.

The five elements retained as central in the reform are shown in Table 5:1,
and will be described, along with the problems they hope to solve.

Making Results the Focus of the System's Objective

The logic of the health-care system is one of developing more and more
services regardless of their relationships to health outcomes. All groups,
including professional associations, established community organizations,
etc., are demanding additional resources to meet this objective. They are not
to be blamed and their intention is laudable, except that it neglects the most
important criterion for providing a service, that is, its contribution to health
improvement. Not considering that result leads to an exaggerated emphasis on
services. There is no limit to the quantity of services to be provided to insure
accessibility to those services and their technical quality except the constraint
of money. The most serious consequence of this approach is that the health-
care sector views itself as a service-production rather than a health-production
system. It tends to forget the contribution of individuals, families, communities and other sectors to health improvement.

Table 5:1. Summary of the analysis of Five Central Elements of the Quebec Health-Care Reform

Problem Identified	Elements of the Reform	Expected Impact	Challenges Conditions of Success or Failure
1. Focus on services and resources not on their impact on health	Result-oriented management and health and welfare policy	• Better basis for decisions concerning allocation of resources and evaluation • Emphasis on prevention • Participation of other sectors	• Grouping of all interventions around objectives • Relationship between resource and achievement of objectives • Organizational obstacles
2. Current financing focuses on the providers of services, not on population needs	Allocation of resources on a population basis and program budgeting	• The budgeting envelope being closed, less incentives for producing services • Providers will settle where the population is because money follows populations	• Criteria for equitable budgets • Method for evaluating performance
3. The ministry is confronted with problems that could be solved at the regional level. Citizens are not involved enough in decision making	Decentralization to regional boards and participation of citizens	• Decisions closer to where action is • Solution better adapted to particularity of the region • Better coordination and cohesio through PROS	• Participation and representativeness of the population • Resistance of the Treasury Department • Universal application
4. Lack of representation of citizens in decision making	Participation of citizens on Board of Directors	• Decision closer to where action is and based on consumers' rather than providers' viewpoint	• Participation • Representativeness
5. Duplication and lack of complementarity between services provided for similar	Unified boards of directors for organizations serving same clientele within a region	• Clientele better served by one or more organizations • Choice of the most appropriate intervention	• Well accepted • Participation of the population is high

In order to focus the system on health and well-being problems, the ministry has just made public a health and well-being policy that sets out:

- objectives centred on the reduction of specific problems and the need of particular clienteles; and

- strategies to be favoured, including the recognition of the essential contribution of individuals, families and communities and other determinants of health.

This document is a main tool for allocating regional budgets, and for evaluating the effectiveness of the system.

Allocating Resources in Terms of the Population to be Served

This element is closely linked with the first. Put together, they constitute the basis of the new philosophy of management that the ministry wants to extend to the whole health-care system from the top level, the ministry, down to the organizations.

Traditionally, budgets have been established from year to year, most often simply indexed without questioning the needs of the clientele and the performance of the organizations. Allocation methods have been based on the provision of services and not on the health and social needs of the population to be served. As a result, the more equipment and providers of services a territory had, the higher the budget it received. It is a resource self-generating system.

The ministry intends to change this method of allocating resources by introducing a combination of zero-based and program budgeting.

The health and well-being policy to which I just referred, is the basis for improving the system of resources allocation. It specifies five program areas:

- social adaptation (child abuse, violence, delinquency, etc.);

- public health;

- physical health (low weight birth, cardio-vascular, cancer, etc.);

- mental health (suicide, depression, etc.); and

- social integration (handicapped persons, old age people, etc.).

Those five areas regroup 19 priority problems identified in the policy document. The budget of the ministry will be organized around these five areas of intervention. Regional boards will be asked to submit to the ministry a service organization plan in each of the five areas (called in French "Plan Regional d'organisation de Service" and abbreviated as PROS).

These plans will identify the needs of the population and the clientele to be served. They will specify the objectives to be pursued and the interventions to be undertaken, by linking all the services rendered to the objectives and the interventions. The regional board will receive its budget from the ministry on the basis of these plans and will redistribute it to organizations and agencies according to the same logic, based on criteria coherent with the plan.

As of now, only regional plans of services for mental health have been elaborated. Eventually, they will extend to all five areas and apply to the whole budget distributed by the ministry to the regions.

Decentralization to Regions by Creating 17 Regional Boards

The 17 regional boards will replace the present 12 regional councils as of October 1992. The idea sustaining decentralization to regions is to bring decision making as close to the action as possible. In addition, citizens will gain more weight in the decision-making process. This is reflected in the structures of the regional board.

First, there is the Regional Assembly, which is composed as follows:

- 40 percent of the members elected by the public and private institutions;

- 20 percent are elected by the community organizations;

- 20 percent are elected by the organizations that the regional board designates as being the most representative of socio-economic groups; and

- 20 percent are elected by municipalities.

The number of members varies according to the size of the region, from 150 in the larger, to 60 in the smaller ones.

At the second level, there is the Board of Directors whose composition is as follows:

- 20 members are elected by the general assembly in the same proportion as above;

- 1 or 3 members appointed by the 20 elected members;[4]

- the chairman of the regional medical commission; and

- the executive director of the regional board

The functions of the Regional Assembly are:

1. To elect every three years the 20 members of the Board of Directors.
2. To designate substitutes for each group of elected members.

3. To approve regional priorities concerning health and social services.
4. To approve the annual report of activities of the regional board.

The specific functions of the Board of Directors and consequently of the regional board are:

1. To insure public participation by seeing that mechanisms for public participation provided for in the Act (e.g., formation of users' committees, supervision of elections and appointments of the members of Board of Directors) are applied.
2. To identify needs and determine priorities regarding health and welfare of its population in order to elaborate service organization plans (PROS).
3. To establish and implement service organization plans; those plans must be approved by the minister.
4. To allocate the budget for the implementation of the regional service organization plans developed for the region.
5. To evaluate the effectiveness of health and social services.
6. To coordinate the work of institutions and community organizations and medical services, particularly in the context of ensuring an equitable distribution of resources through complementarity and shared services.
7. To manage the public health program which is a PROS.
8. To establish a public health department replacing the departments of community health as they now exist.
9. To recommend a public health director to be appointed by the minister.
10. To prepare a regional medical staffing plan based on the organization plan of every institution concerned with the provision of medical services. The plan will be reviewed every three years. It must be submitted to the minister for approval. Once this is done, the regional board approves the organization plans submitted by the institutions.

Board of Directors Consisting for the Most Part of Citizens

This point has been partly covered in the preceding discussion of the regional boards and the composition of its regional assembly and its board of directors. To illustrate further the concern of the ministry with citizen participation, let us look at the situation prevailing before and after reform with respect to the population participation of boards of directors of various organizations and institutions.

As shown in Table 5:2, population representation now constitutes the great majority of members of the boards of directors of the regional boards compared to the regional councils as they existed before reform.

Tables 5:3 and 5:4 show that the population representation on boards of directors has increased not only for regional boards, but also for short-term hospitals, CLSCs, reception centres and even university hospitals.

Table 5:2. *Representation of Citizens on Boards of Directors of Regional Councils and Boards Before and After the Reform*

	Before	After
Municipalities	2	4
Socio-economic groups	3	4
Community organizations	-	4
Board of directors of institutions	-	8
Others	1	1 or 3 (co-opted)
TOTAL	6/15	21/23 or 23/25

Table 5:3. *Citizen Participation on Boards of Directors of Short-Term Care Hospitals Before and After the Reform*

	Before	After
Users' committee	2	2
Socio-economic groups	2	-
Population	-	4
Co-opted members	-	2
TOTAL	4/14	8/17

Table 5:4. *Citizen Participation on Boards of Directors of Various Establishments Before and After the Reform*

	Before	After
CLSCs	7/14	9/15
Reception centres	5/16	9/17
University hospital centres	4/16	8/20

In addition, to ensure that ordinary people be elected as representatives of the population, the Act stipulates that no person employed by the Ministry of Health and Social Services, a regional board, an institution, any other organization providing services related to health and social services or the Health Insurance Board or renumerated by it (e.g., physicians, dentists, etc.) may vote or be elected under the category of representative of the people. Likewise, a person employed by an institution or practising his/her profession in it may be elected as member of the board of directors only in that capacity. In sum, various measures in the Act tend to preserve the prime role played by ordinary people.

Unified Board of Directors Grouping More Than One Establishment

This measure aims to solve some of the problems caused by the lack of complementarity between organizations. A good example of this lack of complementarity is the parallel development of day hospitals and day centres attached to extended care hospitals and reception centres respectively; or that of home-care hospitals and intensive home-care services offered by short-term care hospitals and CLSCs. In sum, it is as if every institution tries to provide all the services to meet all the needs of its clientele.

In response to this problem, the principle for creating a unified board of directors is that organizations located in the same region and serving the same clientele should have the same board of directors. This concerns the following institutions:

- residential and long-term care for the aged and with those less than 50 beds;
- rehabilitation centres for mentally impaired persons;
- rehabilitation centres for persons with hearing impairment;
- rehabilitation centres for persons with visual impairment;
- rehabilitation centres for persons suffering from alcoholism or other problems of addiction; and
- child and youth protection centres and centres for young people and mothers having adjustment problems.

Institutions belonging to each of those categories and located in the same region are grouped under a single board of directors. Obviously, this measure is applied with great flexibility in large regions such as Montreal to take into consideration other factors such as ethnicity or language.

In concrete terms, this means that 666 public organizations will be administered by 477 board of directors, implying that 189 boards will disappear. This is a modest result and there is still room for improvement. But this result shows a promising beginning.

The composition of the boards is inspired by the same principles as those for hospitals, giving a large place to citizen participation. The reaction of the population has been very positive. During the election of May 1992, 180,000 people voted, and 7,000 applied as candidates for only 2,000 positions available. This reflects the interest of people in these matters.

EXPECTED IMPACT OF THE FIVE ELEMENTS OF THE REFORM AND CHALLENGES SPECIFICALLY RELATED TO THEM

The question that can be raised at this point is what is the expected impact of those measures and what challenges are raised by their implementation?

The two last columns in Table 5:1 summarize the different parameters for each of the five elements. We will discuss the expected impact and the challenges for each of the five elements.

Result-Oriented Management

Expected impact

- The establishment of clear and measurable objectives will constitute a sound basis for making choices and decisions concerning the allocation of resources; and for evaluating the effectiveness and efficiency of services.

- It shifts emphasis from curative care to prevention and health promotion because it identifies all interventions related to specific objectives. It is then possible to consider different strategies and choose the most cost-effective one.

- It gives consideration to intervention resorting to sectors other than health. Hence, with that instrument, the Ministry of Health and Social Services and its network can play a pivotal role in promoting intersectorial actions.

Challenges

- Most of the challenges here are technical and methodological. The main question is: Is it possible to group all interventions of the health-care sector around specific objectives? The document presenting the health and welfare policy has made a major contribution in that direction by grouping health and social services around 18 objectives and then into four programs or fields.

- But some objectives are difficult to quantify, particularly those pertaining to the social and welfare domain.

- The link between resources and the degree of achievement of health and welfare objectives is not always easy to make because there are so many confounding factors intervening in that relationship.

- There are also professional and organizational obstacles such as: professionals who are reluctant to see their practices evaluated and especially by outcome-oriented methods; organizations who pursue legitimate goals other than health improvement for their clientele or population; managers of organizations and managers of health-care systems who have a different logic or perspective. The focus of organization is the production of services and the acquisition of resources. It is implicit but not explicit that the organization pursues health objectives. This view is difficult to reconcile with that focusing on health objectives held by managers of systems, territories, regions, or districts.

In sum, the organization perspective and the population perspective are not easily reconcilable in the health-care sector and this calls for management models capable of dealing with complex systems.

Finally, models that make explicit the relationship between resources, services and outcomes, as well as specific outcome indicators have yet to be developed.

Allocation of Resources on a Population Basis and by Program

Expected impact

- Since the budgetary envelope is closed, there are incentives for the managers to reduce or even eliminate inappropriate utilization of services.

- And for providers of services, there are fewer incentives to increase the production of services (analogy with HMOs).

- It creates an incentive for providers of services to settle where the population is; this should favour remote and under-resourced areas, but penalize over-resourced urban regions.

Challenges, obstacles

Here again, challenges are found at the level of methods and tools:

- They concern criteria to be used for establishing an equitable per capita adjusted budget.

- The main question is: What is the basis for adjustment? Criteria will be based on characteristics of the population: age, sex, socio-economic status, health status, etc. But what will be the respective weights of those factors?

- How do we evaluate the performance of a region? Needs and results are measured by the same health indicators. Hence, deterioration of health status over time may be due to a poor performance of the health-care system, but to other factors as well. How do we interpret such results? Do we decrease the budget because of poor performance or do we increase it because of increasing needs?

These are some of the challenges to be faced with allocation of resources based on population needs and by program.

Decentralization to Regional Boards and Increase of the Citizens' Participation or Decision-Making Bodies

Expected impact

- Decisions will be close to where action takes place and, hence, solutions will be found that have a better chance to be adapted to the realities of the region and to be applied.

- Through the regional program of services (PROS) a better coordination and a greater cohesion between services is to be expected.

- All possible advantages linked to decentralization should also apply to health and welfare.

Challenges, obstacles

- Citizen participation is not always easy to obtain. How do we get ordinary people to become interested in management, decision making and in health matters? Representation is a necessary but insufficient condition for ensuring universal participation.

- Representativeness is thus the important issue. How do we make sure that ordinary people are elected and that they can defend the interests of people rather than the interests of particular groups. Safeguards have already been placed in the Act to ensure that ordinary people truly representative of the population get elected. But electoral procedures and regulations have to be refined so that they do not get taken over by particular interest groups.

- Resistance to decentralization comes from many parts. We will return to this more general point later. One important resistance will come from the government's Treasury Department because of the decentralization of the budget and the lack of control, an unusual practice for the Treasury Department.

- Universal application. The regional budget must cover all activities and services within the region. If there are exceptions, such as university hospitals or certain types of programs, the whole system fails because some important elements are not included in the PROS. Hence, the cohesion to which we referred earlier will no longer exist.

The question remains whether it will be possible to include all services and interventions into the PROS. If some organizations happen to escape and obtain their budget directly from the ministry, the system then fails because allocation of resources at the regional level between different strategies will be severely compromised.

Participation of Ordinary Citizens on Board of Directors

Much of this has been discussed in the previous section. The expected impact is to make the views of consumers and ordinary citizens prevail rather than those of providers in the decision making at different levels, including hospitals, CLSCs, etc.

As pointed out earlier, challenges and obstacles here are likely to occur mainly with respect to participation and representativeness of the population.

Unified Boards of Directors for Establishments Serving the Same Clientele

Expected impact

- The different organizations will be forced to adjust their services to the needs of their clientele.

- The clientele will be offered a greater variety of services and hence it will be possible to choose the most appropriate intervention.

Challenges and obstacles

This measure has been widely accepted, except of course by the executive directors who lost their jobs. Participation of the population in the election has been high, as illustrated earlier.

THE CONTEXT OF THE REFORM:
CONDITIONS OF SUCCESS OR FAILURE

Let us now turn to more general contextual conditions that may influence the success or the failure of those five elements of the reform, or of the reform itself.

Before embarking on those questions let me clarify one point. One might argue that the five elements just presented do not correspond to what can be defined as innovations. Indeed, nobody would claim that citizen participation, program planning and budgeting (PPBS), and decentralization to which those five elements relate are new or innovative concepts. Furthermore, experiences reported with respect to those concepts have very often failed to bring about the expected results. Hence, why would it be different with the Quebec health-care reform?

First, the experiences reported elsewhere, specifically in the United States, are not generalizable and do not apply to the Quebec or Canada situation. For instance, Canada compared to the United States, has a very decentralized political system and a different culture.

I do not mean to say that the elements of the reform stem from new and innovative ideas or concepts. What is innovative in the reform is that a provincial government has made a firm commitment to those principles for reforming its health-care system and has used the legislative process to insure that they are implemented. What is innovative is that the concepts of citizen participation, decentralization and program budgeting are put together in a coherent plan for change. Hence, because those concepts are linked together, their interactions add to the potential effect each of them has. For example, program budgeting has a better chance to succeed in the context of decentralization because it gives the ministry a logical and additional method for allocating budgets to the region, based on the needs of the population rather than on those of providers of services.

Now we will turn to the more general contextual factors as they may affect the success or the failure of reform.

Let us begin with citizen participation on boards of directors. This practice has been established for 20 years in Quebec. The experience has been frustrating in many regards, mainly because citizens were largely in the minority on those boards dominated by providers, and too frequently discussions focused on the concerns of service providers. But the tradition of citizen participation is now better established than it was in the early 1970s, when it was initially introduced.

Let me take another example of contextual factors that may create favourable conditions for reform, the population perspective on which program budgeting is based. This approach has been widely adopted in the health-care sector and result-oriented management has been implemented not only in institutions responsible for community and public health, but also in instances having territorial jurisdictions (e.g., regional councils). In fact, the greatest influence that promoters of community health have had in the health-care system may be on the institutions other than community health by proposing methods and techniques that have become integrated in the management of the whole system.

Of course, aside from the favourable conditions, there are also obstacles to overcome. For example, resistance to decentralization will come from many groups, but particularly the provincial centralized organizations such as establishments, organizations, physicians' federations and unions, etc. In this respect, the resistance coming from the government itself must not be underestimated. As a friend of mine used to say, sometimes you wonder if the ministry contributes to the problem rather than to the solution. As mentioned earlier, a strong resistance will particularly come from the Treasury Department and this resistance is likely to introduce rigidity and excessive control and regulation as a great part of the regulatory measures already introduced in the Act to satisfy the Treasury Department's requirements.

Reform has been criticized on many points as being too technocratic, not enough concerned with organizations, and as relying too heavily on the legislative process rather than on the establishment of incentives. Those critiques are probably well founded, but represent more analytical viewpoints than arguments against the reform. It is much easier to criticize a reform than to build it. The government used the main instrument it had for inducing change: legislation. And it is a powerful one, especially if it is coupled with other measures such as introducing financial incentives. Besides, the recourse to legislation does not exclude the possibility of using other measures.

The most important contextual factor, however, remains the funding and financing of the system. A few months ago the minister made public a document on this matter, which clearly stressed the difficult financial situation in which the Quebec government is caught. Of course, all provinces are faced with the same problem. We all sympathize with that, but the tendency is to decrease the governmental contribution to the financing of health care. The document seems to favour the solution of the government's withdrawal from certain programs such as optometric, dental care and other auxiliary services. Recently, the minister announced a cut of $135 million in health expenditure for 1992-93 and of $122 million for 1993-94 as a result of the government withdrawal from certain programs or its limiting financial contribution to health care.

Progressively, the proportion of health-care expenditure assumed by the government will decrease and this may have an influence on the degree of control it exerts on the health-care system and thus on its ability to implement reform. There is evidence that countries with strong public health-care systems have succeeded in better controlling health expenditures. The best example of the extreme and worst position in that respect is the United States with close to 12 percent of its GDP devoted to health-care. As Evans convincingly argued, publicly provided health insurance enables not only risk pooling, which private insurance offers as well, but also redistribution of wealth from lower to higher risk individuals and mechanisms for the collective purchase of health care, and consequently for cost and quality control. Health care has to be provided through a public monopoly so that real cost control can be achieved rather than just cost transfer.

Current measures taken by the Quebec government, and other provinces as well, to reduce its contribution to financing health care is an erosion of this principle and constitutes a slippery slope toward privatization. Such a context creates unfavourable conditions for implementing reform.

CONCLUSION

In concluding, the reform of the Quebec health-care system is now in the process of being implemented according to a three-phased time schedule: first goes from June 1992 to April 1993; the second from April 1993 to April 1995; and the third after 1995.

It is too soon to assess what the final impact of reform will be. But, one effect is already known and should be underscored. The process leading to reform has involved the professionals, the organizations and the people. It has provided an opportunity for exchanging divergent views and for making consensus about others. The dynamic created around that process has had an effect on the attitudes of everyone concerned with health care. They have become more conscious of all the problems identified by the Rochon Commission and by the process that led to reform. It is difficult to put a finger on a specific result of the dynamic created by the reform process, but its pervasive effect will probably make reform more acceptable and easier to implement. Only, however, if the contextual factors to which I have just referred do not create insurmountable obstacles to its implementation.

Notes

The contribution of my colleagues in the preparation of this paper has been important and certainly deserves co-authorship. However, since their formal agreement on the content of the paper has not yet been obtained, I assume the sole responsibility for this paper in its present form.

[1] This section reproduces almost in its entirety a part of the following article submitted for publication: F. Champagne, A.P. Contandriopoulos, J.L. Denis, A. Lemay, R. Pineault. "Options for health system regulation: the case of the Quebec health care reform."

[2] Québec, Commission d'enquête sur la santé et le bien-être social, *Report* (Quebec: Gouvernement du Québec, 1969).

[3] Québec, Commission d'enquête sur les services de santé et les services sociaux, *Report* (Quebec: Gouvernement du Québec, 1988).

[4] Three in Montreal Metropolitan and Monteregie regions; one in the other regions.

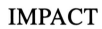

IMPACT

6

A Consumer's Perspective

Joan P.H. Watson

The challenge before us is the re-allocation of health-care resources and the need to look at health in a broader socio-economic context. Can the system cope with an aging population and new technology? What contribution do you expect from consumers?

It is difficult to imagine what our role might be in this. That is not to suggest for a minute that we do not want one. But how does the end user participate in developing healthy public policy? How do we develop and express our vision of what constitutes health? How do consumers get in on the task of setting goals and objectives that will give us a system that is efficacious, caring, and cost efficient? If we refer to the Government of Ontario document *From Vision to Action* produced by the Premier's Council on Health Strategy, we find a vision of health and health goals developed in consultation with consumers.

> We see an Ontario in which people live longer in good health, and disease and disability are progressively reduced. We see people empowered to realize their full health potential through a safe, non-violent environment, adequate income, housing, food and education, and a valued role to play in family, work and the community. We see people having equitable access to affordable and appropriate health services regardless of geography, income, age, gender or cultural background. Finally, we see everyone working together to achieve better health for all.[1]

In pragmatic terms how do we achieve this vision?

The Council set up five goals with very specific and practical objectives and highly innovative approaches to the actual re-allocation of resources.

These documents were accepted in the Legislature after the change of government in 1990. There were 40 people, including the premier and seven cabinet ministers, representatives of all the stakeholders, the clergy, and the public involved. This was a most uncommon group, with a variety of political beliefs — unlikely to reach consensus on anything, unlikely to change their territorial positions. However, over the four years — with a demanding schedule of general and committee meetings — attitudes and convictions did change. Trust developed and a most innovative form of democracy took shape.

Health was addressed in its broadest sense with the involvement of the ministers of COMSOC, Health, the Environment, and Labour; as well as deputies and key bureaucrats as observers. Other than being fed once a day, and having the pleasure of hearing and talking with world-renowned guests, none of us was paid by the Council. That, I think, is important. We were privileged to have an active role in change. These were our objectives;

- To shift the emphasis towards health promotion and disease prevention.

- To foster strong and supportive families and communities.

- To ensure a safe, high quality physical environment.

- To increase the number of years of good health for the citizens of Ontario by reducing illness, disability and premature death.

- To provide accessible, affordable, appropriate health services for all.

For the most part, consumers have allowed themselves to accept a passive role: "whatever you say doctor," which also suggests that we have clung to a medicalized model of health. To paraphrase Dr. Jonathan Miller in *The Body in Question,* when we reach a level of unacceptable discomfort and concern over our health, we decide to become a patient, with an attendant loss of identity and dignity. In the past, we have not perceived ourselves as partners in "sick fix."

On the other hand few health-care professionals perceive us as clients who ultimately pay the bills, albeit, for the most part through taxes. We have abrogated an active role in deciding how we can best be served by the system and the professionals in it. We have been mute about our discontent in the face of what we perceive to be lack of involvement and compassion on the part of some caregivers. We have been passive about a lack of accountability, accessibility and responsiveness on the part of the governments who dole out our dollars.

We are too often fearful and compliant, and simply want to get in and out of the system, unscathed and feeling better, if at all possible. Some consumers still equate health care with sick care. However, more have become conscious of our responsibilities in the promotion of our well-being through healthy lifestyle choices that can delay or even prevent the onset of illness. We also know instinctively that a bad day on the job, or no job at all, makes us feel rotten. We know that a single mother who juggles a job, day care, and an evening of household chores becomes a tired and stressed woman more vulnerable to picking up the cold her child brought home from school. We know that economic circumstances beyond our control — a rent increase, a broken-down car, or not enough money at the end of the week — erodes self-esteem and puts a strain on family relationships. We do not yet have the insight to tote up all these pressures and to assess what impact they might have on family health.

Physicians recognize these stresses, but they cannot relieve them, or, with fee-for-service payment, take the time to address them. With physicians, the emphasis will remain on medical intervention. Dr. Brian Holmes, former chairman of the Ontario Council of Health thinks that typifies the kind of reaction one gets towards prevention. "Curative medicine is much more challenging and interesting," he says. "You can see the results almost right away. With prevention, you might not see any for 25 or 30 years — there's no drama to that." Although the elderly account for 20 percent of all doctor visits, it is still possible to graduate from most medical schools with no exposure to geriatric medicine. Geriatrics is hardly a practice of heroic outcomes. At best it is one of slow progress and yet the population is aging. We need more specialists in geriatrics.

I think a lot of consumers would be surprised and relieved to know that there are thoughtful people who are looking at health outcomes from a much broader perspective. The Canadian Institute for Advanced Research states that: "the dramatic improvements in the health of the average individual have been primarily a result of increased prosperity."[2]

Exactly how this increased prosperity has been translated into improved health is not fully understood. Rich people continue to live longer than poor people, substantially longer. That is not to denigrate the importance of health care. Medical interventions can be decisive for the health or even survival of particular individuals. These advances have permitted the prevention of certain diseases, the cure of others, the mitigation of symptoms of chronic illnesses, the more effective repair of damage from injuries and the rehabilitation of individuals with disabilities.

But it is clear that the determinants of health go far and beyond health care. We are becoming increasingly aware of the limits to what medicine can achieve. That makes sense to the average consumer, particularly if we look at a common scenario that has an impact on a sense of well-being, which is the way many of us think of health: days when we feel good about things generally.

For example, is it possible to feel good if you are a woman in the "sandwich" generation. She runs a household and works at a part-time job. The household consists of a spouse; a frail, elderly parent; and a teenager with a negative attitude towards school and an inclination to resent questions about his friends and outside activities. That woman is not going to have a sense of health and well-being.

The determinants of health include social, economic and cultural factors under the headings of physical environment; family structure; life experiences; situations at home, in the neighbourhood, and at work; as well as psychological factors such as: ambition and motivation; social acceptance or rejection: economic factors related to employment, earnings, housing and income support for vulnerable groups.

If consumers knew that when policymakers talk of re-allocation of resources for the enhancement of family well-being, and addressed these issues, then consumers might feel more optimistic about innovation. But they are also very practical. How long will it take? A whole new approach to healthy public policy is akin to turning a supertanker around at sea. It takes one nautical mile to begin the change of course after the initial command and 15 miles to turn it around 180 degrees. We could wish that this vision of health had translated to action ten years ago.

Consumers are concerned over what they perceive as a general lack of caring in the health-care system. One on one, in their relationships with health-care professionals, they seem to have a greater level of satisfaction, and if not, they are less likely today to put up with what they feel is a callous attitude. They will find someone else. What drives consumers crazy is attempting to get answers from governments on anything from qualifying for drug benefits to finding a nursing home.

CONSUMER WORRIES:

WOMEN: Getting old and being poor and sick.
Getting old and living to see Medicare crumble away.
Losing the family home and life partner.
Becoming dependent on children and losing independence and mobility.
Having no rewarding or relevant role in society.
Having pensions eroded by inflation and taxation.

MEN: Losing the capacity to earn a living.
Having too little pension for comfortable retirement.
Losing home or spouse.
Losing status in a community.

There is a reason why you see a donut shop on every corner. The coffee shop is a highly underrated support system for the vulnerable unemployed male who needs a non-judgemental environment.

While there is government commitment to improve child daycare facilities in Ontario, families in other provinces are dismayed by the federal government's retreat from a national program. What are the opportunities opening up in the field of genetics? Are our fears about genetic engineering legitimate? Who has the ultimate say in how far we go in the area of genetic engineering and identifying predisposition to disease? If it becomes possible to accurately predict the onset in mid-life of a lethal disease, do we really want to live our productive years under the shadow of this knowledge? Will our employer or insurance company have access to the information as well. What are the benefits and dangers of individuals having unique identifiers, numbers that can "spill the beans" on our health history and possible prognosis? This data has great benefits to the planners who want to have systems and services in place to meet the future needs of consumers. But what are the dangers in the loss of privacy to consumers?

Consumers hear about rationing. Who is going to decide whether we can get a kidney transplant or not? If only so many transplants can be done in a year in an institution, who plays God? Does Dr. X get a dozen a year and Dr. Y 14? Is it the doctor or a medical ethics committee who decides a man with two little kids to raise deserves to live, and a 50-year old woman is denied the chance because most of her productivity is behind her? Would it help if we were more generous organ donors — or only add to the cost if procedures are not rationed?

What does it mean when the minister of health says redirection of resources means closing hospital beds in order to improve community health services? If you have a heart attack does that mean you might wind up in the corridor waiting for a bed? And what are these improved community services? Will you be able to go to a nutritionist for an analysis of your dietary habits and get it paid for by Medicare? Can you get your groceries delivered if you are housebound? Will you go to a birthing centre with a midwife instead of a hospital to have your baby? If you do, what happens if you deliver prematurely? Can you talk over your family health concerns with a nurse practitioner instead of a doctor? Consumers perceive nurses as friends. De-institutionalization could also mean dumping Alzheimer patients into communities ill-prepared to cope with them.

What do consumers want? We want reassurance that universal health care will continue, and will provide appropriate services. We want to be partners with health-care professionals and take on a greater role in the decision making that will affect our well-being. I grant you, some people want all the decisions to be made for them. They do not want a negative prognosis. A coping mechanism becomes maintaining hope through ignorance. But that surely, is only the minority. If you opt out of decision making, you do so at your own risk. Dr. Michael Rachlis states that when Canadian doctors treat lung cancer,

> it turns out that many recommend a course of therapy which, according to scientific evidence doesn't work. Even worse, there's some evidence that doctors employ treatments they themselves would refuse if they were the patient in question.[3]

There are several types of lung cancer, over half are non-small cell cancers. The survival rate for this form is grim. Surgery can cure only 5 to 10 percent of patients and over two-thirds of those operated on will actually be worse off after surgery. What's more, no regime of chemotherapy has been found useful for these patients. Yet many Canadians are subjected to the needless misery caused by this aggressive, costly, yet ineffective cancer therapy. The question is why?

Dr. John Evans, past dean of medicine at McMaster University, and former president of the University of Toronto believes that cancer patients are not offered choices about their treatment in an even-handed fashion. "Doctors," he says, "have difficulty holding back even when there's no prospect of a patient benefiting." Most provincial medical associations claim that doctors provide the services patients demand. Dr. Evans disagrees. "We don't have patients calling the shots," he says "Patients are like the shuttles in a badminton game."

That brings us to palliative care — an enlightened approach to the treatment of people whose lives are coming to an end. No amount of sophisticated technology, at whatever expense, will remove the fact — life ends in death. The humane objective is the well-lived life, not the extended death. Palliative care, whether given at home through community services, or in an institution, offers a high quality of life to those for whom quantity is in short supply. If health-care services offer extension of life through the extended preservation of bodies after the minds have gone, or heroic terminal measures which simply add to the pain and distress of patient and family, we may not wish to call these outcomes "health."

Jonathan Swift is believed to have said that "every man desires to live long, but no man wants to be old." On his behalf, I will modify the quote: no woman wants to be old either.

Dr. J. Fraser Mustard, who heads the Canadian Institute for Advanced Research proposes a scenario which he believes we can reach, provided this country can develop appropriate and innovative healthy public policies. He suggests that if we could modify some of the insidious things that erode the health of individuals we might expect that with reasonable good fortune and a fair wind, many of us could reach the fine old age of 85 without experiencing too much disability and illness. Eighty-five would be an attainable biological mark. We would approach it with a vigorous step, and then succumb to a relatively fast, and merciful deterioration. That would save money in the health system. Then we could re-write Jonathan Swift. We could live long, productive satisfying years and bow out with relatively youthful grace.

I used to be very opinionated about quackery and the dollars that consumers spent on dubious health cures. I still do not think much of them, but after all, legitimate doctors use placebos, and who really understands the role of the mind over illness? This was brought home to me when I set out as an investigative journalist to expose phoney cancer treatments being purchased by Canadians for thousands of dollars. I chose two groups to follow. One was located in a group of 20 people from Calgary who paid for treatment in Mexico at the clinic where Steven McQueen eventually died; and the second group, choosing so called alternative medicine, was from Manitoba. They were trekking to Montana to sit below ground in dripping wet abandoned uranium mines to soak up radiation cures. In trying to interview the professed doctors in Mexico and their Canadian clients, I only succeeded in being run out of Tiajuana by the local police and a guard armed with a machine gun.

Montana was much less exciting. After looking at hundreds of letters and testimonials of cures pinned to walls in the mine shaft, I sat freezing on a bench, wrapped in a six dollar Mexican blanket I had bought two days before, listening to ecstatic reports of cures from the cancer patients around me. I followed their progress back in Canada for a year or more and so help me, I could not see any difference in outcome from a similar group taking conventional therapy in Canada — with one exception: they were happier and more optimistic about their futures. I do not know whether they lived any longer but their quality of life was improved. What I had set out to expose had given people hope. I was reluctant to rob them of that.

How we treat the terminally ill and the old is a measure of our nationhood. We cannot reach the point of valuing elders without demonstrating that we also have compassion for the powerless, the immigrants, the single mothers, the poor, the self-abusive, and the lost. I believe a nation can be measured by its attitude and actions towards those with little power. And so, by beginning at the end, caring for the old, we arrive at the beginning: we treat our children as our wealth and our only hope for the future. This principle of compassion works equally well when communicating to people about health. We must meet the needs of individuals — not systems.

At one time, health promotion was seen as something that encouraged people to adopt healthy lifestyles: following nutritional guidelines, having good personal hygiene and being physically fit. Today, health promotion means this and more: we know that inequities in health opportunities are a major issue in health promotion. Everyone's health remains directly related to their economic status. Rich people continue to live longer than poor people, substantially longer. We know affluent people are less likely to make poor food choices, or to smoke. We do not really know why. We do know that when people adopt one healthy behaviour, there is a domino effect: one good habit tends to lead to another. For this reason, there is a vigorous debate over whether we should continue to expand the menu of medically derived interventions, or whether more emphasis should be placed on the role of socio-economic factors that would allow us to better understand the prevention of disease and the promotion of health.

The Canadian Institute for Advanced Research has said:

> If much of medical care is not and in present circumstances cannot be, expected to do much more than mitigate or palliate the course of established illness — lung cancer, for example; or arthritis, or mental illness — then alternative approaches outside the health care system itself may warrant more investigation.

> If technological intervention is of a type which clearly needs the highest level of resources to ensure success, well and good. But if very highly trained and high-priced personnel and/or complex and expensive equipment, are being used to provide 'reassurance to the worried well,' or in circumstances where emotional support by 'informal' caregivers is more appropriate (and as/or more likely to be successful), then the high-priced interventions represent simple waste.[4]

What do consumers want? Do they want generic drugs after a reasonable time for brand-name profit taking? If consumers knew that of the approximately 3,000 drugs regularly prescribed less than half have been tested (by the manufacturers not the government) there would be a call for more stringent regulations. Reputable drugs are often misused. About 20 percent of all hospital admissions of the elderly are caused by toxic reaction to drugs.

Consumers do not want to be kept in the dark. We were incensed to learn that one federal government official wanted the Meme breast implant removed from the market five months before Ottawa gave the device a clean bill of health. That lone voice in the bureaucracy maintained that persistent infections and other severe complications were deemed to outweigh any possible advantage to women. And yet the department chose to go with an evaluation from a plastic surgeon who concluded that the Meme was as safe as any implant on the market. Women have come forward since with horrendous stories of deformity and illness.

Consumers would like to have faith in government regulations and inspection of health devices and medical technology. Instead, we are becoming increasingly disgusted by what we perceive as negligence. How can a heart valve be left on the market and in use for years after it has been identified as having a strut with a failure rate that cries for recall and notification of patients at risk? Consumers want accountability.

Governments and caregivers need to have an ongoing dialogue with users about all the issues. The ability to communicate with individual Canadians begins with showing some comprehension of individual concerns and the impact that government policy unexpectedly has on us. For example, the Province of Ontario made a long overdue analysis of dollars spent on health care for Canadians in the United States. Ontarians had learned that they could by-pass waiting lines to obtain treatment unavailable in Canada and OHIP would pay. In a cost-cutting move, the province severely limited access to U.S. health care under OHIP. However, also caught in the cutback were retired Canadians who traditionally have escaped for part of the winter to a condo-minium or trailer park in Florida. If you believe that having some lifestyle choices to make, that mobility and a change of pace enhances the well-being of the elderly, this would seem a short-sighted move. Perhaps insensitive is a better word. If "Snowbirds" were causing health-care costs to rise signifi-cantly, explaining this to the public would have shown the government in a more sensitive light. However, checking the cost of the health care that these vacationers would have used at home versus the costs while in the United States might have shown that being confined for a winter here produces more disability and resulting costs than having the benefits of a warm climate. The government might save more by investigating why some doctors bring elderly patients back every week when they do not really need to. This was reported by Dr. Dorothy Ley in a study of the elderly for the Canadian Medical Association.

In broadcasting, news and information programming has often been called "public affairs." But when, as an individual you think about it, it is hard to make any connection between public affairs and private concerns. For this reason, as a broadcaster, I seldom thought of the CBC audience of one million, five hundred thousand people as a rippling tide of faces, just out there, somewhere. I always visualized one person in my mind. Someone I felt might use the information I had in order to solve a problem of their own. In my mind, I was never involved in public affairs. All I have ever cared about is the private concerns of individuals.

Whether it is broadcasting or health care, in order to be meaningful you must meet the concerns and, hopefully, the needs of the individual.

This is the challenge. And if we are to try to give Canadians the most appropriate services for the enhancement of health, and the treatment of illness for the $70 billion spent on it each year, we need to involve the individual in the dialogue, the exchange of information, and in the decision-making process that is proceeding today at an accelerating pace as the pressure for change increases. As individuals, we are beginning to relate personal lifestyle with health outcomes. If there are distortions in our perceptions of how health is promoted and care delivered in Ontario among health-care professionals, educators and governments, pity the consumer.

If you are distressed that most of our opinion is shaped by the media, then consider offering some alternatives. Interactive communications by phone, fax, modem, satellite communications and other interactive technology could be employed if people with power had the will to do so. Toronto Hospital does — they say — give power to the patient. The system might end up saving money for the publicly funded health-care system, too, if patients decide they do not need the various operations that doctors order as a matter of routine. Some say it could help deflect rationing.

I admire Professor Deber's respect for the patient as partner. "I would rather have the choices made by the patients based on what they want or need," she says, "I see this as being far preferable to the rationing of care with some bureaucrat making the choices for us." Under the new system, patients watch a video that uses interviews with other patients and medical experts to set out the benefits and risks of conventional surgery and inform the patient of alternative treatments. The video is linked to a computer that provides an individualized assessment, after details of the patient's medical background are entered, and calculates the odds of success and failure. The information is flashed on the screen at key points during the video.[5]

In addition to being able to contact stakeholders and government, consumers need a comprehensive library of health-related information ranging from regulations to community help programs and services, to basic information tapes on health subjects. We need people who answer telephones and are qualified to help find the specific information required. We need more programs such as Toronto's Consumer Health Information Service and Kingston's INFOHEALTH. The information should be in user friendly forms which for some would be hard copy in bold print. For others an audio tape would be more useful. Videos of nursing homes in a catchment area would help consumers find a suitable one, particularly if there were a companion print-out that would give the basics you would expect from any hotel enquiry: facilities, one, two, three or four-star rating, what costs are covered by the system, what upgrades are available and for how much, and when will a bed be available? Often a family is faced overnight with the task of finding an appropriate home for an incapacitated relative. Where do you begin to get information with the same dispatch you can look up data on the best toaster to buy? Or a house? Another example, if there are three treatments for prostate cancer, you should be able to get a tape on the day of diagnosis to give you a synopsis of each procedure, giving benefits and side effects to augment the information given by the physician so that the patient can take some responsibility for making an informed decision about treatment relative to his lifestyle and age.

In the meantime, what we read about most is bed closures, waiting lists for surgery, and turf wars among professionals and institutions all chasing the same dollars. We do not understand the fact that there is an essential threat to universal health care in Canada. Much of the current fiscal distress in provinces across Canada has been triggered by cutbacks in funding from the federal government. Bruce Little, a writer in the field of health economics reminds us that as the *Canada Health Act* stands now, the only way Ottawa can enforce universal Medicare standards is by reducing cash health payments to provinces that violate those standards. Since these payments are declining, so is the control of the federal government.

However, until the slack is out of the system, until governments and providers accept that the information we want is not a rationalization of their own positions but policies that meet our needs, we are going to be a little testy about further taxation — call it user fees or whatever.

Gross mismanagement of the resources we have has been proven — no company would put up with such disregard for inefficiencies, lack of accountability and wastefulness. When resources are redirected and other budgets are cut our question will be: Are these the appropriate changes for the improved health status of Canadians?

Consumers are quite ready to be more responsible for their own state of health.

Behaviour modification has payoffs. Consumers can also pursue other health promoting activities such as keeping a check on blood pressure, or having a pap smear — although the rate of accuracy of these tests is less than reassuring.

If you ask: Are consumers willing to contribute in some measure to the treatments we receive, the answer could be we already do, through one of the highest taxation rates in the world. Well what about a small user fee each time we go to the doctor? Would $5 be reasonable? This is a loaded question — if it is indeed a question at all. If the government decides to go ahead with this, the fee will be implemented like the GST — and somewhat like the GST or the provincial sales tax, or the income surtax, it would be increased at the will of the government, not the public. User fees are unfair — an inconvenience to the affluent; a burden to the poor. I sympathize with the bind that the provinces find themselves in through the cutbacks of transfer payments by the federal government. Consumers know that the squeeze has been put on hospitals to economize, rationalize, regionalize. But as an astute observer put it: the first time you squeeze a soggy sponge — you get a lot of water. The next time you get a dribble, the third time the sponge crumbles.

In any case, we need reassurance that the squeeze is being applied to the most wasteful, inefficient and ineffective elements in the system. We know that there have been sufficient studies done to provide a workable blueprint for appropriate change. We suspect a lot of wasteful practices are being protected. The people who are almost completely excluded from a role in redefining the system are the users. We believe that if consumers were presented with fair alternatives in the pursuit of health for all, we would be allies for innovation.

While consumers would like to have the comfortable good old days back again, we know that change is inevitable and desirable. This is the challenge to both the stakeholders and the powerbrokers: Do you have the courage and political will to adjust your own imperatives, and institute change in the best practical interests of us all?

Notes

[1]Ontario, Premier's Council on Health Strategy, Health Care System Committee, *From Vision to Action* (Toronto: Premier's Council, 1989).

[2]Canadian Institute for Advanced Research, *The Health of Populations and the Program in Population Health* (Toronto: Canadian Institute for Advanced Research, 1989), p. 1.

[3]Rachlis, Michael and Carol Kushner, *Second Opinion: What's Wrong with Canada's Health-Care System and How to Fix it* (Toronto: Collins, 1989), p. 129.

[4]Canadian Institute for Advanced Research, *The Health of Populations*, p. 14.

[5]*Globe and Mail*, Thursday, 30 April 1992, p. A12.

CHALLENGE

7

Reforming Health-Care Financing in the United States

Stephanie Woolhandler

It is fair to say that with the current U.S. health-care system, we are on the brink of financial and moral bankruptcy. Chart 7:1 represents the rising costs in U.S. health care. These costs are going up just as rapidly in 1992 as they were 10, 15 or 20 years ago. Now, of course, the other side of the crisis is the moral bankruptcy over the fact that 35 million Americans are uninsured (Chart 7:2). It is estimated that at least 2 million of these people are uninsured because they are medically uninsurable. Who are medically uninsurable people? Well, if you work for a small company or are self-employed and have health insurance but develop a condition such as diabetes or breast cancer, you will loose your insurance at the end of that benefit year and be unable to purchase insurance at any price. It turns out that 6 percent of the American people have been refused insurance coverage for medical reasons and an additional 7 percent had been told that they were going to be charged a higher rate. Even among the 86 percent of Americans who have some health insurance, vast proportions are only partially insured. There are approximately 15 million Americans with coverage that would leave them bankrupt in the case of a major illness. Some 27 percent of the American population has insurance with a life-time limit of $100,000 or less, so if, for instance, they got a really serious illness they would not be covered. Medicare pays about 50 percent of senior citizens' medical bills, consequently a senior citizen pays more than 18 percent of income for out-of-pocket health-care costs. Ten years ago this was 13

Chart 7:1. *Insurance Overhead as a % of GNP, United States and Canada, 1965-91*

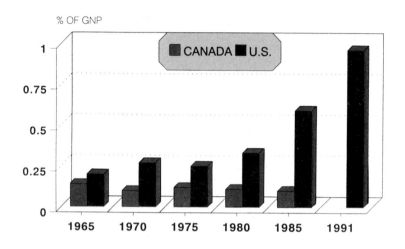

Source: Statistics Canada & NCHS/Commerce.

Chart 7:2. *Number of Uninsured Americans 1976-90*

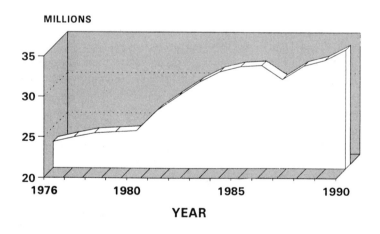

Source: Himmelstein, Woolhandler, Wolfe — Tabulation from CPS & NHIS Data.

percent. Along a similar vein, 5 million young women in the United States of child-bearing age, do not have coverage for maternity costs.

Adults, less than 65 years of age with insurance who had a serious or chronic illness were asked about their access. All have insurance, but it turns out that 12 percent reported a major financial problem due to illness in the past year. Nineteen percent of people with health insurance who had a serious condition, did not see a doctor, 15 percent could not get drugs, physical therapy or other care.

Partial coverage is another aspect of the moral bankruptcy of the current U.S. health-care system. Thirty-eight percent of American people avoided medical care because of its costs in the past year. But the problem is even more severe, Americans who have good coverage are fearful about leaving their jobs, even if they are dissatisfied, or not being fulfilled. When asked: Has anyone in your household ever said they do not want a job because of health coverage?, approximately one-third of middle-income Americans said "yes." People have to keep their jobs in order to keep their insurance.

There is also the phenomenon of welfare-lock, because women on welfare do receive Medicaid, the government financed insurance program, but the low paying jobs that they might take to get off welfare very seldom have health insurance coverage. Many women, particularly if they have children with medical problems, simply cannot afford to take jobs. Of course this is only part of the overall societal crisis in the United States. In the last decade the United States is virtually alone among the developed world in seeing an actual decrease in real wages.

Finally, despite this, American workers work more than those of any other nation, with the average American worker having fewer than 11 paid vacation days per year. Canadians are not doing much better at slightly under 15; Japan, the United Kingdom, Germany and Holland all have over 24 days of paid vacation. Now what happens to someone who is uninsured or underinsured who shows up at a hospital emergency room. There is the example of an unfortunate woman who was hit by a truck when she was walking along the road. Her chart reads: "Twenty-one year old female in motor vehicle accident last night, seen at Washington Hospital (a private hospital) and transferred here, a public hospital, secondary to no insurance." The rest of the chart continued with descriptions of multiple broken bones, pelvic and rib fractures; her blood count fell from 37 percent to 27 percent despite the transfusion of 2 units of blood, indicating severe internal haemorrhage. Nonetheless because she flunked the wallet biopsy, because she did not have money nor an insurance card in her wallet, she was placed in an ambulance without a doctor or a nurse in attendance, and transferred nearly 30 miles to a public hospital. That is why I recommend that if you come to the United States for a visit you buy yourself a very expensive pair of Gucci loafers. Now you may feel ridiculous going on vacation in expensive loafers, but if you are unfortunate enough to be mugged and your wallet is stolen and you end up in an emergency room comatose and with no identification, the loafers will help people assume you are insured and you may avoid what happened to that woman. In fact it happens 300,000 times each year in the United States — a patient appears in an emergency room urgently ill and is turned away because they are uninsured or underinsured.

But even these dramatic cases in emergency rooms are only the tip of the iceberg of unmet medical needs. There is also the question of preventive care activities such as pap smears, blood pressure tests, or breast examinations. A nationwide study was done some years ago on American women. It turned out that the lack of health insurance was the most important predictor of failure to receive needed preventive care, a predictor that was actually strengthened after multi-variant statistical control for comfounding factors such as income, urban and rural residents. Similarly, if we look at rates of prenatal care for the disadvantaged, we see actual deterioration. There is data for black women who had no prenatal care before the third trimester of pregnancies, from 1970 to 1988. In the early 1970s we saw just what we in the health-care field like to see, steady improvement, a steady decline of indicators of ill health. But beginning about 1980 there has been actual deterioration in access to this important preventive service. In a similar pattern there were mortality rate improvements in the 1960s and 1970s but, beginning about 1980 total stagnation developed, a failure to see any improvement in the health-care indicators in the past decade.

The United States has dismal health statistics, we have one of the highest infant mortality rates in the developed world. Canada is somewhat better but not as good as a number of the Scandinavian countries. When we compare the survival of a man born in Harlem in New York City, with the survival of a man born in Bangladesh (Chart 7:3), in fact the survival in Harlem is worse. For females, the numbers are about as high in Harlem as in Bangladesh. When we look at the causes of this excess death in the African American population, we find that the deaths are due to things like cardiovascular disease, cancer, infant mortality or diabetes. In fact, the excess deaths in our disadvantaged populations is due to things that medical care can do something about.

To summarize, in the United States in 1992 about one-third of Americans are inadequately insured — either uninsured or partially covered. They are often denied care, and they are sicker and die younger than the affluent and well-insured.

Now this would be a tragic necessity if the United States had a shortage of medical resources. But at this point, one in every three hospital beds is lying empty, and we hear of an impending surplus of physicians and other medical

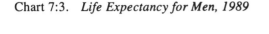

Chart 7:3. *Life Expectancy for Men, 1989*

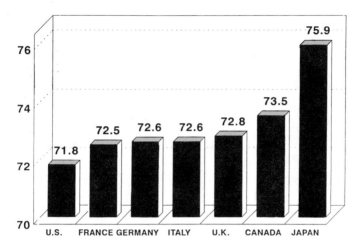

Source: OECD, 1991.

personnel. But, of course, there are problems with having an excess or surplus of resources. There is an old saying that when you go around with a hammer in your hand, pretty soon everything starts to look like a nail. We have a tremendous problem with excess surgery in the United States. It is estimated that at least 10 percent of all surgery done is unnecessary. For some surgery the rates of unnecessary procedures are higher.

In the case of coronary artery bypass grafting, a team of experts from the Rand Corporation reviewed the charts from a random sample of U.S. hospitals that perform the surgery. In 14 percent of all cases of coronary artery bypass graft, the surgery was clearly inappropriate and in another 30 percent, the indications for surgery were equivocal. The inappropriate group actually contained six charts of patients who had had coronary artery bypass grafts, *while they had clean coronaries,* zero percent stenosis, absolutely normal heart and coronary arteries. The situation was even worse when the Rand researchers looked at carotid endarterectomy, a surgery that cleans out arteries in the neck — only one-third were clearly appropriate. Surgeries such as hysterectomies, and Caesarean sections have tremendous excess rates of operations. Such surgery not only does no good, but can harm the patient.

Chart 7:4. *Appropriateness of CABG and Carotid Endarterectomy in U.S.*

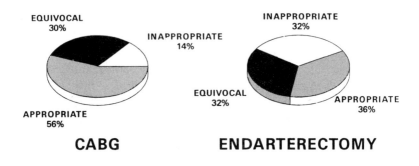

CABG   **ENDARTERECTOMY**

Source: Rand Corp., Jama 260:505 & NEJM 318.721.

Similarly, when we look at the question of duplication of technology, there are other ways that excessive technology and excessive investment can worsen the quality of care. Hospitals that do fewer than 200 cardiovascular operations per year have higher death rates than high volume hospitals. Their death rates are about one-third to two-thirds higher than high-volume hospitals. Of California hospitals doing open heart surgery, more than one-third have a dangerously low volumes and produce a higher death rate and higher costs. Similarly in Des Moines Iowa, population 380,000, there are two hospitals doing renal transplants. One did 8 cases last year, one did 15. A hospital 100 miles away did 69 cases. The duplication of technology actually is driving down the quality of care delivered in the United States and is clearly raising costs. Competition is defined by multiple hospitals in a market area. Therefore, the more competition there is in a market area (the more hospitals there are) the higher the average costs.

In the United States today, we are rationing in the face of a surplus. Now as I remember Economics 101 from college, you are supposed to ration a shortage, yet in the United States we are rationing health care in the face of 300,000 empty hospital beds; in the face of a growing surplus of physicians; and in the face of millions of unnecessary operations each year. Now, of course, it is difficult when on the one hand there is a patient with no insurance down in the emergency room who needs care. There is an empty bed sitting upstairs waiting for a well-insured patient. It takes a great deal of work to keep needy patients out of empty beds. That in some ways explains Chart 7:5. The number of health administrators is growing at a phenomenal rate in the United States, five or six times as fast as the rate for physicians.

Now to return to Canada and the relevance of the U.S. experience to Canada and vice versa. You are probably aware of an incredible misinformation campaign that is being launched in the United States against the Canadian health-care system. Many in the United States believe that we may need to put an army on our border to prevent all of those Canadians from running across to get to the U.S. health-care system. You would certainly believe that if you listened to the political leadership (political leadership is, of course, the ultimate oxymoron). Paul Tsongas, when running for the democratic nomination for President actually stood up at a press conference and said, "I am a bone marrow transplant recipient. If I lived in Canada I would have died

Chart 7:5. *Growth of Physicians and Administrators, 1970-87 (1970 = 1)*

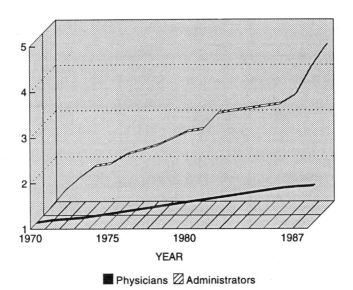

Source: Rand Corp., Jama 260:505 & NEJM 318.721.

because they don't have bone marrow transplants in Canada." Tsongas is supposed to be intelligent and educated. Similarly Newt Gingrich went on National TV and said (Gingrich is a key Republicans spokesman) if you are a Canadian and over the age of 55 with renal failure, you cannot get dialysis, they just let you die. People — including the leadership — go around saying incredibly stupid things like that.

In fact, Canadians do receive more medical services on the average than their American counterparts. Canadians use more physicians, (Chart 7:6) receive more procedures and have more physician's services. For better for worse they also receive more days in the hospital (Chart 7:7). When we look at certain high technology procedures such as transplants, Canadians receive more transplants than Americans (Chart 7:8). Canada does do somewhat more heart and lung transplants, although this figure is distorted by the high number of lung transplants in Toronto, where there is a medical centre. Nonetheless when Americans see this, they are shocked because they have been told by their political leadership that this cannot be true. Of course, there is a cost differential in the two countries, that Canada spends approximately 40 percent less on a per capita basis than we do in the U.S. on health care. You may be less aware of the fact that there is a divergence in the costs for the United States and Canada as expressed by a proportion of GNP. The divergence occurs

Chart 7:6. *Physician Visits Per Capita, 1987*

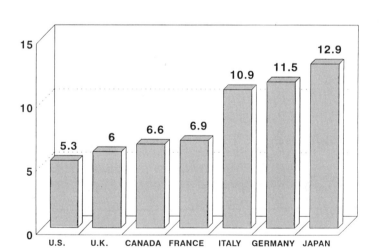

Source: OECD, 1991.

Chart 7:7. *Average Length of Stay in Hospital,*
Patient Days Per Admission, 1987

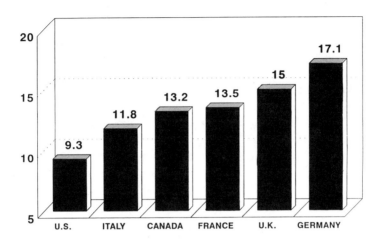

Source: OECD, 1991.

Chart 7:8. *Transplants, United States and Canada, 1988,*
Transplants Per 100,000 Population

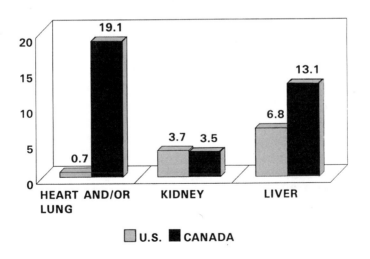

Source: OECD 1991.

precisely at the point where Canada enacted the National Health Program. In the words of Robert Evans, the relationship between universal coverage and cost control is not coincidental, but is causal (See Chart 7:9).

The other rumour that is going around the United States (including the editorial pages in the *New York Times*) is that Canadian health-care costs are actually rising more rapidly than those in the United States. It is unbelievable, that the editorial board of the *New York Times* is saying this. Finally, Canada has been more successful in getting college students to enter medical schools. There is something of a crisis in medical education in the United States as young college students, understandably fearful about making such a major investment in medical school, go into other careers (Chart 7:10).

Now I want to discuss the German health-care system. At this point in the United States the forces that are opposed to a Canadian national health-care insurance system have said that we do not need a Canadian model, but can have a West German model. That is the buzzword on Capital Hill; "We want a West German model, we don't want a Canadian model." Of course there are a number of problems with the West German model: mediocre health statistics (they are not as good as Canada's); and the fact that they employ very few health-care workers (Chart 7:11) — that is how they contain costs. They pay their health workers quite a bit less than workers are paid in the United States

Chart 7:9. *Health Costs as % of GNP: United States and Canada, 1960-91*

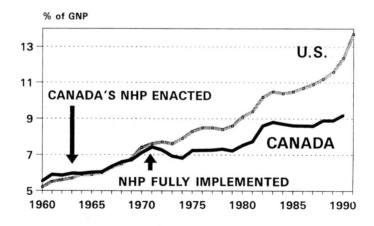

Source: Statistics Canada & NCHS/Commerce Department.

Chart 7:10. *Applicants Per Medical School Place,
United States and Canada*

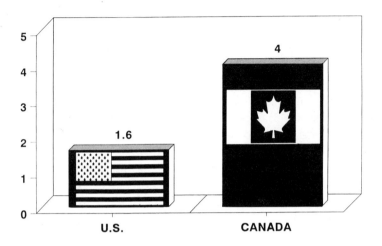

Source: NEJM 1990 322:562.

Chart 7:11. *Number of Hospital Workers Per Bed
United States, Canada, Germany, 1987*

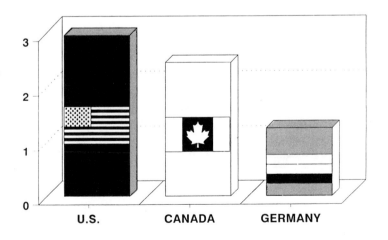

Source: OECD, 1991.

(See Chart 7:12). Therefore, I would think the German model is not very realistic, nobody really thinks we could cut health worker's salaries by 30 percent or lay half of them off. Germany is becoming a buzzword to prevent people from thinking in an open-minded way about what we might be able to learn from the Canadian example.

One of the hottest issues on Capital Hill is administrative costs. It turns out that approximately half of the total difference in health-care costs between the United States and Canada is accounted for by your lower paperwork. In the United States, 24 cents of every hospital dollar goes for billing-related paperwork (Chart 7:13). How can we spend so much money on paperwork? One aspect is our insurance overhead. But with 1,500 different insurance companies billing and literally millions of different patients who have to receive bills, the insurance overheads alone — just the cost of running the insurance system — are extremely high in the United States. They account for about 14 percent of total private health insurance premiums. What is noteworthy is that both Germany and the Netherlands have multiple payer systems, even though they have national health insurance (Chart 7:14). Germany has approximately 2,000 sickness funds, the numbers in the Netherlands are in the hundreds. Multiple payer systems cannot get the type of administrative efficiency that you have been able to get in Canada with a single payer system.

Chart 7:12. *Health Workers' Earnings as a Percent of Average Earnings, Germany and United States, 1970-89*

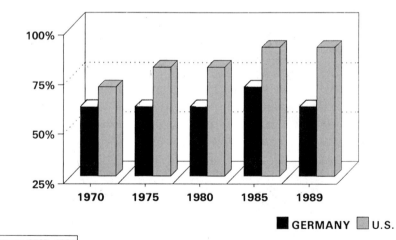

Source: OECD, 1991.

Source: OECD, 1991.

Chart 7:13. *Paperwork Costs, United States and Canada*
A Bigger Slice of a Bigger Pie

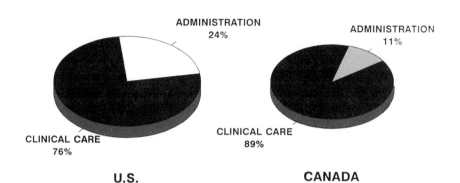

Source: Woolhandler & Himmelstein NEJM 1991; 324:1253.

Chart 7:14. *Insurance Overhead, 1990: United States,*
Germany, Netherlands and Canada

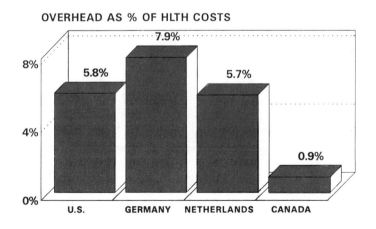

Source: OECD/Statistics Canada/NCHS.

I note a lot of interest in HMOs. There is a belief in the United States that HMOs have got to be much more efficient than other types of health care. But if we look at the administrative side of things, at the insurance overheads of HMOs, private U.S. insurers, and the Canada National Health Program, we find that HMOs are no more efficient than U.S. private insurers, and both are much less efficient than your National Health Program in Canada (Chart 7:15). Your private insurers in Canada have similar overhead costs to U.S. insurers, about 11 percent overhead, meaning you pay them a dollar and you get back 89 cents for care. One example is a managed care program in New Jersey — Prudential Insurance — which covered 110,000 enrollees. In order to run the managed care network, they have 18 nurse reviewers, who review every hospital admission, over the telephone; five physician reviewers who oversee the nurse reviewers; eight provider recruiters who call up doctors and try to get them to sign up; 15 sales representatives, who go around to companies to recruit enrollees from the employees; 27 service representatives who have to deal with all of the irate enrollees who call up and say "Why wasn't my surgery covered?" and over 100 clerks. Managed care creates a tremendous amount of bureaucracy, and any savings that you get out of a managed care system are offset by this bureaucracy.

Chart 7:15. *The Rise of For-Profit HMOs, For-Profits as % of New HMOs, by Year Started*

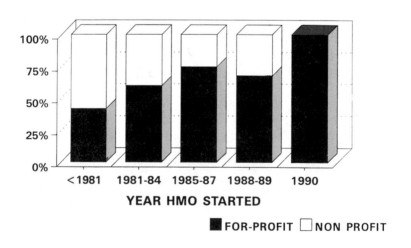

Source: Marion Managed Care Digest, 1990.

As I mentioned earlier, it would be bad enough if the insurance companies only created their own paperwork, but they force tremendous amounts of paperwork on providers. The nurses are required to keep track of everything used by a patient: every bottle of intravenous fluid, the tubing and even the two ounce bottle of shampoo. The nurse must place every billing tag on the patient's chart, when she has the time; and that chart then goes down into the basement of the hospital where all of these little numbers on these billing tags are typed into the computer. The computer puts out a 27-page bill, and passes it on to the insurance company; a portion of the bill goes to the secondary insurer and a portion goes to the patient. A tremendous amount of time and money are wasted on the provider's side. At our Massachusetts General Hospital in Boston, there are about 900 tertiary care beds and over 300 billing staff, a multi-million dollar billing computer, actually a separate building for the billing department. Now you have to compare that to the billing department at Toronto General Hospital, which is a comparable hospital and has half-a-dozen billing personnel Chart 7:16). There is a tremendous amount of money wasted on the provider side.

Chart 7:16.   *Hospital Billing and Administration,*
              United States and Canada, 1987

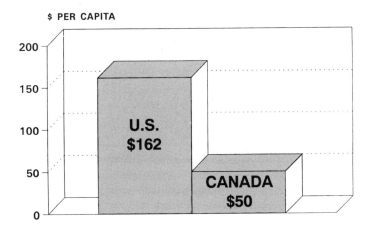

Source: Woolhandler and Himmelstein NEJM 1991; 324:1253.

Now if we look at what is happening in terms of hospital employment over the last six years, it turns out that the growth in employment has all been under the administrative and marketing side with very little growth in professional nursing and nurses aides (Chart 7:17). Of course this is part of a more general social trend that the United States and Canada unfortunately share, we have a tremendous number of managers and administrators, compared to other countries. Finally, who actually pays for health care in the United States? Chart 7:18 divides the U.S. population into income deciles; and then the share of the health payments divided by the share of income for each decile is graphed on this chart. It turns out that the poorest decile in the United States pays more than three times as much of their income for health care, as the richest decile. This arises since our employer-based system is very regressive, since in an employment-based system such as we have in the United States the $3,000 individual policy is, in effect, deducted from the pay of each worker for health insurance. The same $3,000 applies to my secretary as applies to me. More dramatically, the same $3,000 deduction applies to a steel worker who earns $25,000 a year and the chairman of a company who earns $1.5 million. For that reason providing health insurance through employment on a premium basis is highly regressive. But that is what we do in the United States. Now if you have a government-funded system, you at least have the possibility of financing your system more progressively, as is true for the provincial portion of payment in the province of Alberta (Chart 7:19).

Chart 7:17. *% Change in Hospital Employment, 1983-89, by Occupation*

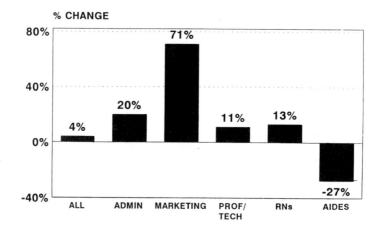

Source: Monthly Labor Review, 1991.

Chart 7:18. *Who Pays for Health Care?*
the Regressivity of U.S. Health Financing

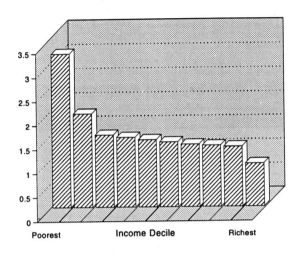

Source: *Oxford Rev. Econ. Pol*, 1989; 5(1):89.

Chart 7:19. *Who Pays for Canada's NHP? Province of Alberta*

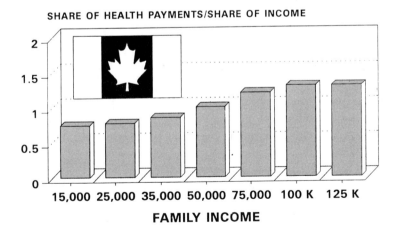

Source: Premier's Comm on Future of Hlth, Excludes out-of-pocket costs.

So in the United States, a movement has begun to grow for a national health program. Many of us are looking to some of the successes in the Canadian model. Not that we want to repeat your mistakes, we just want to repeat your successes. I know my Canadian friends always call me and tell me Canada has this problem and that problem, and I say to them, I wish we in the U.S. had your problems. I am a founder of an organization called Physicians for a National Health Program which now has nearly 5,000 physician members. We are one of the fastest growing medical organizations in the United States. When we first got started a number of people were very sceptical including one editorialist who quipped "Physicians for a National Health Program is a little like furriers for animal rights." Nonetheless, the lesson we think should be learned from the Canadian experience is that we need a national health program that is universal and comprehensive. One that has no out-of-pocket payments; where hospitals are paid "lump-sum" operating budgets — global budgets, where capital budgets are separated from operating budgets; where there is a single public payer; and where we would have public accountability, but with a tendency to minimize bureaucracy. Those are essential elements of the Canadian national health program that Physicians for a National Health Program feel should be adopted and incorporated into any health reform in the United States.

What happens if you ask the American people if they would prefer a system like that? The Harris Poll asked Americans the following question: "in the Canadian System of national health insurance, the government pays most of the cost of health care for everyone out of taxes, and the government sets all fees charged by doctors and hospitals. Under the Canadian system people can choose their own doctors and hospitals. On balance, would you prefer the Canadian System or the system we have here in the United States?" I think that is a pretty fair description of your system. It turns out that 61 percent of Americans were quite sure that they would prefer a Canadian system (See Chart 7:20).

Now this was not that surprising to me, but I know many health policy people were surprised because, of course, the rumour in the United States is that Canadians are totally different from Americans and your health system would never work in this country. All of the Washington pundits from Louis Sullivan, Secretary of Health and Human Resources, and all the way down, know that Canadians are just different. The joke is that Canadians say, "thank you" to the cash machines. But of course when someone actually tried to be scientific about it and asked Canadians and Americans for their views of health care, it turns out we have almost identical social ethics on health care (Chart 7:21). For instance the majority in both countries say that we need one-class care; a tiny minority think the sick should be paying more; majorities think

Chart 7:20.   *Would Americans Prefer the Canadian NHP?*

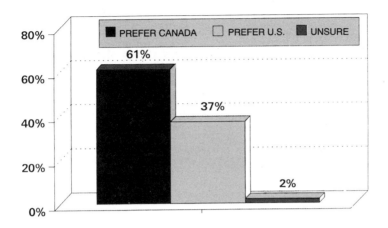

Source: Blendon, Hlth Mgt Q 1989(1):1.

Chart 7:21.   *Americans and Canadians: A Similar Social Ethic*

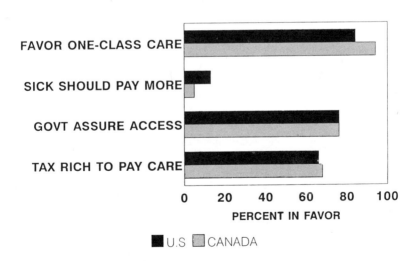

Source: Hlth Mgt Q 1991 (3):2.

the government should assure access; and the wealthy should be taxed in order to pay for care. The social ethics are similar in both countries. Again we look at the profile of the typical American who prefers the Canadian health system:

Table 7:1:   *Preference for a Canadian-Style System by Demographic Group, United States, 1988*

Whites	61%
African-Americans	61%
Hispanics	62%
Executives	67%
White Collar	59%
Blue Collar	60%
Low Income	58%
Middle Income	68%
High Income	56%
Americans who now have health insurance	62%
Americans with no health insurance	61%

Source: HLTH Affairs, 1989, 8(1):154.

I do feelCanadians could be doing more to assure quality.

Finally, I suggest that you could do more, in terms of community input and community control. There is a model in the United States of Community Utility Boards that are actually citizens' groups that monitor utility rates and the location of utility plants. They have their own independent financing to hire economists and experts who advise them so that citizens have a real input, they can have an intellectual input from the independence of providers. We have never done it in the United States for anything but utilities but that is a model I would like to see tried for health care.

8

View from the Ontario
Ministry of Health

Michael Decter

As a provincial Deputy Minister of Health attending the rather historic meeting of health and finance ministers — federal, provincial and territorial — on 18 June 1992 was, as always, a bit of an emotional roller coaster. I am tempted in the continuity with Dickens as our literary reference, to drift towards the quotation of thinking of my role as "the far, far better thing I do than I have ever done before, to the far, far better place I go than I have been before" and also James Baldwin commented for many of us, "the future is like heaven, we like the idea but we just don't want to go there right away."

There were certainly moments during the meeting, as we watched the rather lively debate between M. Bouchard, the federal minister and Marc Yvon Côté, the Quebec minister, when one had a sense that "this is the way the world ends — not with a bang but with a whimper" might be a phrase one could attach. I came away with, I think perhaps, more mixed emotions than my federal colleague although I think she did an excellent job of sketching the background and the history. I think we are in times that have both great opportunity and great peril.

There is a very old story about federal-provincial relations that some of you have heard before and hopefully will tolerate. It is the story of the newly-elected premier of a small and usually un-named province who was confronted his first night on the job by a visit from his predecessor. There was a knock on the door and he was surprised to find the former premier there, they had not really spoken since the election. The former premier thrust three envelopes into the hand of the newly-elected premier and said, "this is all of the advice I have for you," and then headed off down the hall.

The newly-elected premier, filled with the spirit of the newness and the great promises he has made in opposition, thinking that the previous fellow was obviously defeated because he did everything wrong, throws these envelopes into the drawer and gives them no further thought until a few months later when things are not going very well. He is in his office one night having a large scotch and contemplating how little fun it is to be a premier in this particular small un-named province and he comes upon these envelopes.

He opens the first one that simply says, "BLAME ME!" He goes out the next morning and blames his predecessor for everything, the fiscal situation, all unpopular policies; all of it is the fault of the previous government. This works marvelously well, the newspaper headlines are "Mess Found," and "Previous Government Responsible" and so on. This works for 18 months and finally one day, someone at a press conference says to the premier, "Well surely everything couldn't be their fault?" I thought of this yesterday when Don Mazankowski was explaining the inherited fiscal crisis after nine years.

At a certain point this blaming of predecessors does not work very well and the premier, now older and wiser, paws through his desk drawer and finds the next envelope and opens it. It reads "Blame The Federal Government." Well this works really well! He gets re-elected, everything is the fault of the federal government, with the problem in health care being because they have not provided sufficient money; even the disappearance of the fish from his province is somehow linked to the federal government's failure in international affairs. In any event, after being successfully re-elected on a "stand-up for un-named small province ticket," the premier eventually is confronted by reviews expressed by the media and others that the federal government cannot conceivably be responsible and blamed for everything. He retreats to his office and pulls out the third envelope and in it is a small card that simply reads "PREPARE THREE ENVELOPES!"

Federal-Provincial Relations

What was enormously hopeful about the meeting of Finance and Health was the absence of finger pointing and what gives me some hope was that although people went through their set pieces about inherited fiscal situations and on the provincial side, *Canada Health Act* requirements, without adequate stable funding, there was no sense of that being where they wanted it left. There was no sense on the part of any of the parties that they wanted to score political points and avoid trying to find some resolution of the substantive problems. Substantive problems are very real. Both levels of government, the federal government, and the provincial government now have significant structural deficits.

There is, as often said, only one group of taxpayers — us — and therefore the magic solution to find significantly more revenue is not really there. I guess another dimension of this is the emergence of not one but two coalitions, the Coalition to Keep Medicare Healthy, largely spear-headed by the Canadian Union of Public Employees with some 400,000 members, (100,000 of whom work in health care) and the HEAL coalition, with some 500,000 members (largely providers, although the consumer association is part of that coalition). Let me divert for a minute to talk about how those two coalitions see the debate because I think it has become a more complicated and healthier debate than simply the two levels of government arguing about whose fault it is and who is going to have to change in order to fix it.

The Coalition To Keep Medicare Healthy has a seven-point plan. This coalition really has its roots in hospital worker's unions, and feels that we need to:

1. stop the fee-for-service treadmill;
2. give non-physician staff a larger role in patient care;
3. eliminate health care for profit;
4. elect hospital boards as democratized health-care institutions;
5. reduce dependency on prescription drugs and make them more afford-able;
6. guarantee that health care is of the highest quality, whether it is provided in the home, the community or an institution; and
7. encourage preventive care.

The HEAL group have ten principle goals; and they have three specific requests to ministers at this point in time. One is to ensure that consultations with consumers and providers in developing health goals are meaningful and occur at earlier opportunities, so they want to be involved. Two is to establish a stable financial planning horizon, consider transition funding, inviting HEAL to participate in the forthcoming review of major federal transfers to the provinces; and finally, to establish a national task force to clarify the five Medicare criteria and develop more effective methods to ensure their attainment. HEAL and the coalition met with five of the provincial ministers, so we have not yet advanced to the point where it was possible to get 13 governments to agree on which of the two groups or none or both, to hear and the stalemate produced was such that I believe that federal ministers met with HEAL separately and provincial ministers met with each of the two groups, so we are not quite all at the same table yet, but there is some movement in that direction.

The most profound thing that is going on can be summed up in two dimensions. One, everybody agrees that the status quo is not on, that we are in a period of change. Two, everybody puts the umbrellas of health-care reform and quality over the changes that are taking place, although there is fundamental disagreement inside that umbrella about what we mean by health-care reform. Meanings are not necessarily diametrically opposed but certainly when you listen to the prescriptions of the Coalition to Keep Medicare Healthy and the prescriptions of HEAL, they diverge fairly significantly. It is understandable that provider organizations which are largely what the two coalitions represent are concerned to protect the interests of their constituent members. I think it is fair to say that the national organizations have embraced change at the level of their statements, speeches and policies rather more generously than their provincial constituent organizations. I think that is understandable. It is not the federal minister that gets up to explain why a certain procedure is not being performed or why a certain patient is leaving the country, it is the ten provincial and two territorial ministers that have the privilege. As Nye Bevan once said of the National Health Service in England when he introduced it: "if a ward nurse dropped a bed pan in a public hospital anywhere in England, the sound resonated through the Parliament of Westminister." I think it is very true that the complaints department for the health-care system that we have is very much the provincial legislature and has its own peculiar dimension to it.

The preparation for the meeting and the document that will result represents very significant intergovernmental work, both federal and provincial, and among health officials to converge what is going on in the 12 jurisdictions. What is going on in each area is not identical; each jurisdiction has its own unique history, differing structures, and relationships.

Underneath the umbrella of the *Canada Health Act* exist a wide range of somewhat misunderstood programs that get called Medicare by the public and are prized enormously by Canadians as constituting one of our unique and distinct differences. One of the difficulties for managers and ministers is that there is a misunderstanding about the scope of the *Canada Health Act*. The *Canada Health Act* starts with a very broad preamble that I believe anyone, no matter how critical they are of the current delivery system, would embrace in terms of the broad health goals and the determinants of the health approach. It then narrows considerably in terms of what it actually provides as core, mandated, insured services. Those services are generally speaking, hospital in-patient services, hospital out-patient services and physician services. The rest of what we can look at as our benefit package, our entitlement package, province by province — be it access to drug plans, access to other providers such as physiotherapists, chiropractors or a myriad of other delivery organizations, community health centres or health service organizations — all of that is well outside the scope of the *Canada Health Act*. All of that is a result of provincial governments spending resources in ways that they see to be sensible investments in health care. Nevertheless, the public view is that this is one seamless system and that any impediment to access of a financial sort or a quantity sort is the erosion of Medicare.

The dilemma for ministers is how to square the circle. I think Quebec is coming to it more directly than the other provinces for a couple of reasons. They started earlier, Quebec amalgamated its health and social services in the 1960s and that move was led by two extraordinary individuals — the late René Lévesque and Eric Kierans, who were twin ministers for that process. As a consequence, almost 30 years later, Quebec is further along and is having more difficulties with the narrowness of what is insured under the *Canada Health Act* and M. Côté was very direct about this. It was a pleasure to have him there since Quebec has not attended any meetings since the failure of the Meech Lake Accord, other than their finance minister who has a mandate to attend if Quebec's financial situation is at stake. The appearance of the health minister and finance minister and relative officials coming back to the table on this issue underscores the extent to which, while Quebec is distinct and different in many ways, health care and the reform of the system is at the top of their agenda.

Quebec has talked about introducing, but has not done so yet, the $5 fee for emergency room service. The case made by their officials was that they have CLSCs, which are really community-based care services. The availability of these services, in their view, meets the test of the *Canada Health Act*; and if someone who does not need emergency room treatment decides that they want to go to the emergency room rather than going to the CLSC, the government feels that it is, under the *Canada Health Act*, allowed to levy a deterrent fee to push patients to alternative services. Now the Government of Canada does not agree with that view and has expressed that opinion directly. That gives you some idea of the complexity of the debate. The dilemma, too, for ministers, is that many of them fear the erosion of the *Canada Health Act* and that any movement towards greater flexibility runs the risk of the complete erosion of the original principles. So you have the province that is probably furthest along in fundamental reform coming up against the narrowness of what is insured.

There is a growing recognition that the narrow investment in physician and hospital services has run its course in terms of remaining simultaneously an important element of health-care delivery, but really not being a place where we are going to see significant gains in terms of health status for the population. As you try and shift the structure of the system, you run up against the anomalies of having part of it insured and part of it discretionary. For example, if you are in a hospital bed, all of your drug costs are covered; however, in

Ontario if you are not on social assistance and you are not over 65 and you are not covered by a private plan, a drug that might keep you out of the hospital is something you are going to have to pay for out of your own pocket. So we have these anomalies as we attempt to shift from in-patient to out-patient, to community situations. That is not actually how the money flows.

Affordability

What you are hearing from ministers collectively, I think, can be summarized in two ways: first, there is now a sixth principle of the *Canada Health Act* stating "affordability"; and that affordability principle is what finance ministers have drawn the line on and said essentially, with the support of every cabinet in this country, that the total provincial budget for health care is enough. There is no evidence to suggest that throwing more money in at this point would achieve any better health outcome although it may buy more services, and therefore health ministers may figure out a way of living within this envelope of affordability. That decision has taken different forms in different provinces and has come at different times. Ontario has come late to the party, not intellectually because intellectually that view has been here since John Evans and Robert Spasoff and others for over a decade, but in terms of the ministry and the government adopting broad health goals and beginning to bring down the growth rate in expenditures that started in the 1991 budget and has continued in the 1992 budget. As I say, Ontario came late to the affordability question and I think it is fair to say that we have all known intellectually that health-care reform was going to be tackled. As with many things in life, it was not until we were forced fiscally to make some changes that we got more serious about them. So we have talked a better game in this country on health-care reform, and I think that is changing dramatically.

National Action Plan

What provinces are finding in the national action plan on physician resources is that much of what we do is both politically and managerially more acceptable and more readily achieved if it is done in a concerted way. There is no point in only one province reducing medical school enrolments when we have interprovincial mobility of physicians. It is really not a very helpful move. An earlier question asked: "Is it very useful if we have international mobility of physicians, that we in Canada restrict or reduce our enrolments?" The answer is we do not have unrestricted mobility of physicians. We do have a court decision that states very plainly in Ontario, that there is no constitutional right to practise medicine and I believe you will see parallel restrictions. The Banff

Communiqué and subsequent work does see a balanced program of reductions in enrolments in Canada and reductions of migration of physicians into the country. Within that, many us are struggling to prevent what I would term "Fortress Ontario." I think that medicine in Canada is one of our unifying forces because of the mobility that is there and I know that it imposes a cost. We tend to pick up a lot of physicians and that costs. The Newfoundland minister recently stated that Newfoundland had lost half of its graduate physicians to Ontario over the last decade and this is putting some real stress on services in the province. But the kind of balkanization you get with provincial credentialism is, to me, not a unifying force in the country, so we are trying to work nationally on this issue and it is squarely on the agenda for ministers and national groups. I think you will see subsequent actions on utilization management, appropriateness and effectiveness.

Basic Questions

These things get jumbled together by ministers but essentially the questions are: What services are being delivered in Canada? What are the specific medical services? What do we know about their effectiveness? and What do we know about outcomes?

> In attempting to arrive at the truth I have applied everywhere for information, but in scarcely an instance have I been able to obtain hospital records fit for any purposes of comparison. If they could be obtained they would enable us to decide many other questions beside the one alluded to. They would show subscribers how their money was being spent, what amount of good was really being done with it, or whether the money was not doing mischief rather than good.

For anyone who thinks that might have been the minister or I on a bad day, that was Florence Nightingale in 1863. Nearly 130 years later I think it is fair to say that many of us in the health-policy field yearn for a day when we could get better comparisons of records and better comparisons of outcomes across even the institutions of our own province, let alone the country.

There was approval by ministers for the creation of a national Institute for Health Information which will build on some existing infrastructure and really try to bring together under one roof, the HMRI, some of the federal work and some other activities. If it is done carefully, because many of us have come to depend at the provincial level on certain data sets that we cannot afford to lose, I think it should go some distance towards Florence Nightingale's quest of 130 years ago.

Quality

Quality Assurance, Total Quality Management, Continuous Quality Improvement — We have all been confronted with various incarnations of the quality
movement. It represents in Ontario, and nationally, one of the interestingly
bright spots in the current reform activity. First, there is good evidence at a
micro-level that quality has not been an overwhelming driver of activity in the
system; that history has — that quality in terms of process has not. Second,
there are some marvellous examples across Ontario of individual hospitals that
have embarked on intensive quality initiatives in seeing quality improved,
costs fall and that is encouraging to everyone involved with hospital management. In terms of the national strategy, I think it is fair to say that we are still
looking more at putting together all of the good evidence from across the
country and all of the good experiences in sharing it, rather than launching
some new quest for some new variation on the quality theme. The issue is
dissemination and application of quality techniques within hospitals and other
health-care provision systems rather than inventing something new at this
point.

There is also discussion of a national pharmaceutical strategy.

Of the major elements, the one that is largely outside the *Canada Health
Act* but has the fastest growth rate of any expenditure are the drug plans. In
Ontario's case, the last decade has seen a 19.5 percent annual increase in the
cost of the drug plan and with heroic efforts this year, heroic in the sense of
unpopular and not well received, we will only be able to bring that increase
down to something in the order of 12 or 13 percent, that is with a 2 percent
price ceiling on existing drugs. The real drivers have been eligibility, utilization and the price of new drugs entering the system. There is a double-edged
sword here, since it is very clear that one of the reasons we can reduce the
scale of our hospital system and reduce the number of beds is that there are
many conditions which used to require surgery, that are now treated with drug
therapies. So, one positive aspect of the continuing ingenuity of the researchers and pharmaceutical and pharmacological fields has been some positive
impact. On the other hand the cost-driver effect is profound and unrelenting;
and we are, in terms of Ontario, at the start of a two-year reform of our own
program.

Ontario remains now the only province in the country that does not have a
fee of some sort or a co-payment on the plan. Quebec was the second-last
province in that regard and they are in the process of putting through a
co-payment. That I guess has not given offence in most of the other provinces
because co-payments were part of the schemes when they were brought in and
so there was a public acceptance from day one. As you would gather it is very

hard in a province where there has been no fee to impose one because it is very hard to distinguish between a $5 co-payment on the drug plan, which would be well within the *Canada Health Act,* and a $5 co-payment on a visit to a doctor which would be a clear violation of the Act. For the rational citizen, it does seem to amount to the same thing, so we have that anomaly to live with.

From Insured Services to Managed Services

Let me turn now from the drug plan to some of the other things that we are doing in Ontario. After comparing ourselves with others across the country, we found that what we are doing here is similar to what is being done in other provinces. There are some peculiar timing and policy variances, but the major thrusts are first of all a shift from an insurance model to a planned and managed system. The role of government was to insure and fund and that role has proven to not have, although it has public popularity, any assurance from ministers of health in this province that they are getting very good outcomes or very good value for the money. So that shift is fundamental.

Physician Services

Let me discuss the implications of that for physician services. Ontario has gone the route of agreeing with its physicians through their organization, the Ontario Medical Association to create a joint management committee for the 30 percent of our total health budget that is physician fees — some $4 billion this year. Under the joint management committee we have created an Institute for Clinical Evaluative Sciences to look at, and bring together a group of leading experts in fields such as clinical epidemiology, to actually look at what we are getting and what are the outcomes of these various procedures.

Our sense was, and I would give enormous credit to the late Dr. Adam Linton, who brought the Ontario Medical Association around, that war was very expensive for both the profession and the government because it prevents either the government or the profession getting on with some constructive work around outcomes and around applying the best knowledge to the practice of medicine. Adam Linton also held very strongly to the view that neither the profession nor the government could do it alone, that the profession lacked the will and the government lacked the credibility. For government to proclaim that this or that procedure was appropriate or not appropriate would drift it into the role of endeavouring to practise medicine which is a very dangerous role for any government or state to be in. It would lack credibility with the public because it would be seen as being fiscally driven, concerned only with saving money. On the other hand, the profession lacks the will to tackle its own outliers because there was really, in an open-ended insurance system, no incentive for the profession to incur the wrath of individuals or the minority by participating in a process that might cause them to have to change their behaviour or to lose income. The rather difficult agreement that was patched together between the government and the profession has, as I think any good partnership has, both risks and rewards for both parties and time will tell how well it works out.

So far we are seeing much more of an engagement by the profession in questions of outcome and utilization. The institute is new, it has been active for a few months, but it will take some time. My own conviction is that this is the sensible way of going about it, that it is the road that offers the most promise of permanent improvement in the quality of those services.

Hospitals

Look at your hospital system. The government has set out some planning guidelines as of January 1993 and we look to moving the provincial hospital system from an average of 1,050 bed days per 1,000 population. That is a consumption number not a capacity number. The old kind of capacity number was for beds per thousand and the problem with the capacity number is it does not reward efficiency — just build the plant and wait for people to go through it. Our belief is that 850, which will represent a 15 percent reduction, is a number that the system can live with. Our evidence, two-fold, is that there are counties in the province where we are seeing hospitals deliver quality care and use something on the order of 700 bed days per thousand, so there are certainly examples where less than that bed capacity is working. There are American examples and one is always careful about transporting experience across national borders because there are important cultural differences. But there are American HMOs that are viewed as well-managed, that are getting by with 450 to 500 bed days per thousand. So 850, in our view, is not an ambitious target and we will probably achieve it in many parts of the province within 18 months to three years.

It also comes very much to the question of capital planning and not building hospitals or hospital additions that are going to be vacant because of changes in technology, changes in our ability to deliver care on an out-patient basis. Now in many cases, they are very controversial because commitments have been made in this province over past decades by various health ministers and first ministers to communities about "the new hospital." So we have all sorts of situations where we favour amalgamation in the community, or role sorting such as the two acute care hospitals in Guelph, where Mr. Blundell has secured agreement that one will become a long-term care facility and the other will remain an acute care hospital.

We have other communities where we have had proposals for amalgamation but accompanied by enormous expansions in proposed service levels that are not within our guidelines. So we have a lot of work to do at the community level and much of it is not readily done by government. Government can set out guidelines, it can set out policies, but for communities, I think we are seeing the unfolding of a very interesting success story across the province. Communities are going to have to roll up their sleeves and hospitals are going to have to work with community providers. The referees in this game are the District Health Councils. When one picks some organization one always makes a choice, not a perfect choice in any sense, some of the District Health Councils are well regarded, have a long history and have done a marvellous job of bringing together various hospitals to plan rationalization of services. But some of the others, such as the Metro Toronto District Health Council are up against staggering scale questions and staggering differences among the types of hospitals that exist on their piece of geography.

But overall, and I would take this as evidence of creativity on the part of hospital managers and boards and diligent work by District Health Councils, the Ontario Hospital Association predicted 13,000 layoffs across the province in the hospital sector. The Council of Health Care Unions went one better and predicted 14,000 layoffs, as a result of funding decisions. They also requested another $600 million from government. That money was not forthcoming, the Ontario Hospital Association met my minister and the premier and said that they would not ask for more funds in fiscal year 1992/93. They understood the government's situation, they would manage within the funds.

They also asked that we jointly talk about how the layoff numbers are but a fraction of what the forecasts were. That is not, in my view, because of bad homework by the OHA, one could have stacked the funding numbers against the pressures from the hospitals and come easily to those numbers. Now the ministry came to slightly lower numbers from that but what has happened, I believe, is a lot of hard work inside the hospital community to find economies to redeploy workers to do some very creative human resource management. The best numbers we have, and they are not easy numbers to get, but we did put $30 million into a Hospital Training Adjustment Program to re-skill workers so that they could move to jobs either outside hospitals or in other hospitals. They have surveyed all of the hospitals in this province, some 2,300 positions have been eliminated but only 400-500 actual human beings are out of jobs because many of those positions were vacant or were simply not refilled. Now no one likes to be in the position of being responsible for one person losing a job let along 400-500, but that in 140,000 hospital workers is a much different number. It is also the case that there will be 2,600 retirements this year from the hospitals, so there is some scope for management.

I go into some detail on this for several reasons. In many communities in the province, a hospital bed has been equated with health-care services. People know how profoundly that delinking has moved over the past number of years. That many services that used to require an in-patient stay are now done on an out-patient basis. There is still more possibilities as we lag the Americans in moving to out-patient care. With adequate follow-up and home-care support and other necessary things we still have some considerable scope there. So we need to shift the debate. The Alberta minister, Nancy Betkowski, said something I considered quite accurate and also quite interesting. I asked her how it was going, and she said, "well, I have the public on the side of reform, I now have the providers on-side with reform, the only people I yet have to convince are my caucus." My minister has many visits from her caucus colleagues who say "yes, yes I agree with all that health-care reform stuff, now where is the new wing for the hospital in community X?"

I think, quite frankly, because of the enormous regard and role of hospitals in communities, particularly smaller communities (it is one of the few remaining social institutions that brings together health care, which is on the top of most lists, and a number of the leading citizens from other walks of life, business, law or whatever as board members) they have a major employment impact. In many small communities, the hospital is the largest employer and has grown and been stable for over 30 years.

You put all of these together and I think you can see that there is a formidable coalition, only part of which is related to the actual delivery of care. There is a kind of Gordian knot of care and employment and income which is very potent in political terms and which we need to carefully undo and we need to do a lot of education as we move through that process. To simply say to people, "well the hospital is not really health care," is of very little value because they say quite rightly, "when my child has a high fever at two in the morning, that hospital emergency room had better be there or you are failing." So we are going through a transition in thinking. One of the agreements, as ministers, is to work out a way of speaking more directly to the public about appropriate use of the health system. This has been the demand from providers for some time, they say in a variety of ways, "why blame us? We are out there doing our jobs providing care and when some 40-year old comes into my office and wants to be tested every week for his cholesterol level, and I tell him that is nonsense, he simply goes down the hall to another doctor until he finds one who is willing to test for his cholesterol level every week." That kind of consumer — as mad shopper, unreasonable, unfettered, sort of maniac out there in the health supermarket — is a view that most providers have. When you say that is 1 percent of the people that come through your door, or 10 or 50 percent you get some variance in view. That makes many providers, particularly physicians, think about deterrent fees and ways of deterring people. All of the evidence says that deterrent fees do not deflect people on the basis of the appropriateness of their use, they deter people on the size of their pocket books and that is not what we want to do.

On the other hand, I believe it is time for government and providers to explain directly, such as a national television advertising campaign, to the people of the country some facts about what is appropriate and what is not appropriate. We have in this province something called the annual health examination. We are the only province that still has one in its schedule of benefits and this is a dilemma. The examination sounds great. Most people say, "well an annual health exam, that's preventive, that's the good thing." So de-insuring the annual health exam would be an act of heroism for any minister of health. On the other hand, when one talks to physicians, they say several things. Many annual health exams are not done for health reasons, they are done because the summer camp requires it, or the employer requires it, or the insurer requires it. So it is not being done either on a treatment basis or on a health prevention basis, it is being done because some third party wants it done. So the issue is, should the government, all of us, pay for those health exams or should the parents of the kids who are going to camp? Oddly enough they do not require check-ups to go to school, and they are at school for nine months and they are only at camp for three weeks. This might seem like an odd choice.

Could we replace this with something better? Could we replace it with a new and improved protocol on health examinations? Could we, for example, say we are not going to pay for an annual health exam for everyone, since we now pay for about a million of them a year at about $40 each. We are talking about $40 million and that is not small change. Another issue is the removal of tattoos. We now pay about $200,000 per year for this procedure.

We have asked the institute to see if they can put together (based on the best existing knowledge out there) some alternatives. Maybe we could say to the public, we believe women of a certain age should have a routine breast screening. They should also have at a certain age, pap tests. Maybe it is worthwhile to have certain tests done on most of us at some point in our life. Maybe there is a new and improved package that makes much more sense in health terms than the annual health exam. But it brings to mind the dilemma we face about going out and saying to the public, without an alternative, that we are de-insuring the annual health exam. We would undoubtedly have our offices ringed with protestors. We know that we are still going to have to pay for some of these extraordinary procedures whose outcomes are dubious.

There may be room here to work with the profession and that is why I think it is important that we are sitting at the table having a rational discussion. To say, well if you are getting a health exam for a third party, we are willing to let doctors bill that third party, we are even willing to help them bill, because that does not strike us as being an insured service. The *Canada Health Act* does not say, thou shalt pay for health exams for summer camp. In the same way it does not say, although it may be of a better value if it did, that we will pay health club memberships. There is an enormous investment by the public in their own health that falls outside the *Canada Health Act*. That is an example of one of the things that we are going to have to wrestle with. There is no big cure, there is no single thing that any government is going to do that is going to fix the system. What we have ahead of us in the 1990s is a lot of sleeves rolled up, hard work on many micro issues of management, of outcome, of appropriateness. Am I at the end of the day an optimist? Yes, I am on what I have seen. I have seen in the short time that I have been in this job an extraordinary change in attitude.

My orthopaedic surgeon father, twenty-five years ago fought a major battle because in those days, in the hospital where he worked, there was a rigid rule that no patient over 70 years of age would be given an anaesthetic. That was the rule. So if you were 72 years of age and you broke a hip, you were not getting that hip repaired. We have come a long way since then. But I say that to gently remind people that we are not moving from an era or a history, where everything was infinitely available where there were no difficult choices, where there were no rules. We are going through an evolution.

We had a period in the 1970s and 1980s of rather buoyant economic growth, rather favourable commodity prices as a country, and rather unlimited growth in health spending. That was not unlimited growth because we could afford it forever, it was unlimited growth because ministers believed that health increasing its share from 10 percent of the budget to 33 percent was the right thing to do. We have now a more mature system. We have made a lot of investments in health-care providers, in facilities, in technologies and now we have an enormous task of managing them better and I think it is achievable. It is not going to be easy, there will be plenty of times when mistakes are made and the ministry will do its share of that and will continue to do its share.

We are working inside a framework of goals and principles; and the goals are those adopted and proposed by the Premier's Council on Health, Well-Being and Social Justice, and Health Strategy and I think there are solid determinants of health goals. The principles are for improved system management to ensure effective use of scarce resources, ensure that all planning and service delivery in ministry programs is done on a basis of reliable needs-based population health data and analysis. We are going to try and drive this thing off at the epidemiology point, not history and politics and attain the highest possible quality of service and ensure that at every level, through consumer and worker involvement, appropriate accountability mechanisms are built in to every program. The issues of accountability, quality improvement, management and collaboration and planning are going to be central whether it is the reform of the *Public Hospital Act*, the reform of the drug program, or changes in physician services. They are reasonable principles, but they will be given life by a lot of individual action, a lot of individual policy decisions over a period of time.

I will not lean on the, "may we live in interesting times" approach because it is so true. Let me go on to something that Chou En Lai said. He was asked, I believe on the 200th or 250th anniversary of the French Revolution how he felt as the leader of the most populous country on earth about it and he contemplated the question and said, "well, it's really too early to tell." That was the same answer I was given one summer ago in China when I asked how they felt about the Communist revolution. They told me that little story and they all laughed politely. Medicare as we understand it in this country is still a very new initiative. Insurance of hospitals happened in the late 1950s, early 1960s and physician services in the late 1960s, early 1970s were still within the previous generation. My late father was a pre-Medicare doctor who was completely entranced with the idea that he would now get paid for everything he did and that the patient did not have to come up with a contribution. He felt that that was marvellous. My younger brother is a physician, post-Medicare physician, who is much more concerned with the percentage increase that is afforded annually and since he has never had to ask a patient for a payment in his entire life, he cannot imagine that such a thing could ever exist.

Lots of things may exist. It will not be any easier to bring about reform in health and health care than it was to move forward and create something in the first place. I think that as a Canadian, it is one of things we are proudest of. Dr. Kitchen, the finance minister from Newfoundland, after listening to health ministers preface everything they said by "of course, we have the best health-care system in the world," finally in a drawled Newfoundland way, began his remarks by saying, "if this is the best health-care system in the world I sure don't want to see the worst." But amidst all of the things that we need to work on and change, I do believe that we all ought to be quite grateful that we are citizens of this country, but we do have a lot of work ahead of us.

9

Rapporteur's Remarks

Raisa Deber

The theme of the conference was Health Care: Innovation, Impact and Challenge. I agree with Dr. Marshall that pursuing this historic challenge is probably an appropriate thing to do. We know what the challenges are. They were reviewed by Amelita Armit, by Michael Decter and by myself. The nice thing about commenting is that I do not have to make any nasty remarks about my own talk.

There is also the backdrop of news stories coming from the recent Ottawa meeting between the federal and provincial health ministers, which is likely to influence the future shape of health care. We heard about some innovations, but in light of the news stories we start wondering, "are we rearranging the deck chairs on the Titanic, or maybe on the Lusitania?"

The innovations shown at this conference are pointing in different directions. Some of them are pure research and may eventually be important, but in the current situation, they are just backdrop. Some of them looked at things such as increased effectiveness, so we saw many pilot projects for service delivery. There were optimistic developments, including technology assessment. Mrs. Armit points out that there is an agreement, and that more emphasis should be put on it. There are guidelines. At this conference I saw several regional programs, including a lithotripsy program, which are trying to develop the idea that we should more effective in how we handle things. There was a very interesting assortment of projects directed towards more consumer education, including a library-based information centre, a diabetes education program, and the work I am doing with Dr. Wennberg with interactive video discs. All of these ideas suggest that we can have shared decision making with informed patients. We kept hearing the word "empower" and it was interesting to me, for I think the word was being used in a lot of different ways and they may not be compatible with each other. There was some confusion between the public as a consumer, a customer, or a patient — whatever word you want to affix — and the public as a citizen. One example was a very interesting presentation of smart cards which talked about empowerment. It meant this it in the sense that a better provision of information could lead to better communication which could then lead to technically better treatment. I think this is something that could be extremely important.

I do not tend to go off to the doctor a great deal, which I rationalize by noting that if we are going to preach appropriate care, we should not keep running off to the doctor. And I have this post-nasal drip that, every year, I let turn into pneumonia and than I have to go and see the doctor and get an antibiotic. This year, I was coughing so much that my husband told me that if I kept him up one more night, the divorce court might be an alternative. So we decided that we had better do something about this cough and the doctor gave me a cough medicine. I took one teaspoon of the cough medicine and could not get up the next day nor the day after that. I was knocked for a loop. I was told that "yes, this is an occasional rare reaction to this particular medication," and upon thinking about it, I realized that I had also had a similar reaction to that medication in a different form when I was in high school. That one I remember, because I passed out in the basement of Simpson's and the sales clerk insisted I go to another department because he did not want the responsibility for anyone passing out in his department. So the smart card technology might have had the ability to record these types of things and would mean that I would not have been prescribed that drug again. On the other hand, it still fits into a pretty passive role for the patient. That is not really empowerment, it is better care and more appropriate care. The other sense we were getting was that the public is being put democratically in control, as shown in the very interesting talk of Dr. Pineault on public participation. As a sardonic political scientist, I then start wondering how we define "the public."

Among the innovations that had a booth was a project called "Health 2000," which was a participatory health study funded by the Premier's Council Innovation Fund. They state that they focus on small communities that report their own health, assisted by professional assessment, with local prescriptions to alleviate problems. I started wondering what would happen if the community did not want to agree with the professional assessors who tell them how they should be thinking. There was also the multicultural community project to assist in placing ethnic community members on health and social service boards. This is an appropriate matter, but you again wonder who is going to come out and want to be on those boards, and is that the public? Indeed, is that even the multicultural public? I am less sanguine about these reforms because one of the classic findings in political science is that people have lives, and they tend not to want to participate in most things. There are too many things going on in life, and you cannot participate in everything. It is the fantasy of Ross Perot's that you can turn everything into electronic voting on all issues, and presumably you are going to know enough about each one of those issues. Those of you on the District Health Council know that the pile of papers you hand your volunteers on any issue is just enormous. It takes a great deal of time and a lot of effort. You say, "why would you do it?" The reason is that you really care about an issue. However, you are particularly likely to care about a health issue either because you make your income out of providing it, or because you receive one heck of a lot of those services. The technical term is that "concentrated interests" are more likely to participate than are "diffused interests." Ordinary people are not as likely to get involved in the health-care system unless they get sick, and then they want to make sure that the services they need are provided, possibly more than "community needs" might warrant. There are some political science studies that have the disquieting finding that communities that became very sensitive to participation turned out to be less sensitive to the wishes of their community because the groups that participated were sufficiently skewed in terms of their wishes and viewpoints. What a politician should be doing is going out and talking to constituents and the community. There is a sense that the process gets short-circuited, and you end up with less, not more, responsiveness by government. That is the worry I have.

I also think there is a myth of the "community," in that people have different interests. People do not all want the same things, think the same way, or believe in the same things. Yet we talk about "the community" as though it is monolithic. It is the idea of the New England town meeting — there are 27 of us and we all come together in the town meeting hall and decide how we are going to run things. I notice that very few of those models apply to Toronto. Greater Toronto has about 4 million people in it. So we keep worrying about Toronto later and we solve Fort Frances. But at some point we have to figure out what we are going to do about Toronto.

So I guess I am wondering whether we really know who our customers are, because there is another set of trends that are being seen in the innovations, and that is to increase government control at the same time as we decrease government contributions. Now as the federal government would testify, this is a really neat trick, if you can bring it off. Mr. Decter noted the fundamental shift which is happening between an insurance model and a planned and managed system. At some fundamental level, there may be a contradiction between this and patient empowerment because of the difference between meeting patient demands, having patients define what they want and meeting patient needs. Needs are not defined by patients; needs are defined by some type of expert or another, not by the people who receive the service. To me the Oregon experience, which is being held up as a model of citizen participation, is precisely the opposite, because you are not defining it for yourself. Instead, one group defines the needs of others. If it involves citizens, you have to be bound by the decisions you are making. If we are talking of needs assessment, in most cases we do not think we are going to be bound. We think we are making these rules for others, usually the poor. We think we can obtain better services if we need them for ourselves. So I look at some of the innovations and I see a danger that some of them may hurt our system, rather than help it.

Dr. Woolhandler made us feel much better about Canada's system. The nice thing about looking at the U.S. system is that anything looks good by comparison. I certainly see why the insurance industry loves the American system. But then I start looking at some of the reforms that we are discussing, and I wonder if we are bringing in some of the same problems. She talked about the essentials of our system and stressed things such as universal comprehensive coverage, no out-of-pocket payments, hospitals being paid lump-sum global operating budgets, separate capital budgets, the single public payer, public accountability and minimal bureaucracy. Then I look at innovations like Resource Intensity Weights and Case Mix Funding and other types of global activities. I look at regional budgets with chargebacks from one institution to another when you serve patients who are coming from somebody's else catchment area. I wonder if we are putting in some of the complexities when the saving glory of our system is that we have not had them. Now I know that this is heresy to administrators who think that these sorts of things are wonderful, but I would want to take a careful look at the sort of information systems that we are going to need. If the information system is to improve quality of care and appropriateness, great. If it is just to try and figure out how much nursing and laundry is taken for a particular Resource Intensity Weight, so that you can try and get your global budget adjusted — I am not as convinced. And if it is to shift expensive patients elsewhere, or to move marginal but profitable care, it could be harmful.

Dr. Pineault noted that publicly funded mechanisms are better for cost and quality control, otherwise, what you start getting into is cost transfers. He is a little worried that Quebec may be making a mistake in opening the door for cost transfers. I liked the metaphor that Dr. Marshall used of a blind driver heading for the wall. My query is: Do reforms in some areas get in the way of others? There are some obvious examples. Health does not exist in a vacuum. One example of a policy process which may have unintended effects is constitutional change and what any changes may do to health care. But there are a whole lot of others we could look at. Mr. Decter mentioned drug policy

— it evokes the question of making trade-offs between what the trade needs are and what the health policy and affordable care needs are. Dr. Woolhandler mentioned the underuse of non-physician personnel. One of the things I have been wondering is what happens if we take the concept of pay equity to its logical conclusion, and what then happens to labour substitution. Because if somebody is doing the same job as a substitute, should they not be getting the same money? But if they should be getting the same money, what do we need to substitute for? There seem to be certain fundamental contradictions that we have not sorted out yet, but we are stuck with an agreed-upon policy of raising the salaries of lower paid workers. I have heard rumours, for example, that someone has decided that mid-wives, when they come into the system, should get $100,000 per year. If you compare them with doctors, that may sound reasonable. If you compare them with nurses, it may sound less reasonable. We keep talking about moving into the community, but we do not pay the same money in the community. So if we are going to move people from institutions into the community sector, are we going to increase salaries from the community sector to the same level as institutional salaries? If we do that, our savings are going to evaporate pretty quickly.

As well, there is the whole question around regionalization. I believe in rationalization of services. I believe in capped budgets. But some of the ways we are looking at regionalization, and I take Quebec as a particular model, suggests to me that we are ignoring some of the major technological trends. Advances in communications technology imply that you could have a Centre of Excellence in an institution serving local clinics, with the local doctor's office allowing patients to receive care in their own community with expert advice from the central Centre of Excellence. There are many procedures where we do not need to have the patient in the same room as the doctor. As we start moving to minimal invasive technologies and other things like that, the patient and the provider are going to have to be physically together less and less often. Yet we are making resource management plans and budgeting plans on the assumption that it is going to be other way, and that we are going to have to start decentralizing care to each of the regions serving people. This may be remarkably ineffective, from both cost and quality standpoints.

I was very encouraged to hear Mr. Decter's statement that he does not see a single cure for the system — he sees a lot of hard work and he emphasizes quality and appropriateness. He also noted that there is no evidence that putting more money into the curative system leads to better outcomes. He is clearly right. If I can be a little heretical, since health promotion is the new religion, I am going to play devil's advocate and suggest that there is also no evidence that putting more money into social welfare-based prevention leads to a better outcome. In fact there is no evidence that money into any of these things will have any impact at all. I am not sure if we know any way to prevent family violence, I am not sure whether we know of any way — AIDS prevention or no AIDS prevention — to stop adolescents from having sex, or to stop adolescents from driving too fast. So will the money buy results? Some of the arguments seem as irrational to me as the current set of feminist demands that we spend in proportion to burden of illness, rather than spending in proportion to our ability to get pay-off. So the argument is "breast cancer is killing a lot of women, ergo we have to spend so much on breast cancer" and if you say, "well, ok, but do we know how to prevent or even cure breast cancer?" — the advocates do not care. They look at how much is spent on AIDS and suggest that spending for breast cancer has to be proportionate. However, if we are going to spend based on burden of illness, rather than based on ability to buy the desired outcomes, we are going to be in the same type of mess as we were in with a system based on ability to buy hospital beds rather than impact on outcomes.

I also have a moral question: Do people really want the "nanny" state? President Havel of Czechoslovakia has been making some very moving statements about the futility of leading. He disagrees with the notion that we can improve human nature by government fiat and points to a whole series of field experiments which seem to prove his point. Then I looked at the pamphlet that the Premier's Council on Health, Well-being and Social Justice distributed. They first state that they have a vision of health — this is from the old Premier's Council, which did not much care yet about well-being or social justice, just health — and they had their vision of health.

> We see an Ontario in which people live longer in good health, and disease and disability are progressively reduced. We see people empowered to realize their full health potential in a safe non-violent environment, adequate income, housing, food and education and a valued role to play in family work and the community. We see people having equitable access to affordable and appropriate health care regardless of geography, income, age, gender or cultural background. Finally we see everyone working together to achieve better health for all.

Now, that is pretty ambitious. They then went from there to a series of health goals. I then looked at the new vision. Our new Council has a vision of social justice.

> We see an Ontario where people value the dignity and self-worth of individuals, where systematic discrimination and barriers are eliminated and where society celebrates human diversity and strives towards common purpose. We believe that a socially just community supports and expects a balance between individual and collective rights and responsibilities. We see an Ontario in which everyone has a fair chance to achieve economic, social and personal well-being. We believe that individuals and groups can realize their potential and achieve social justice

through full access to the determinants of health which enhance well-being and through active participation and community life. We believe that resources must be equitably distributed. Policy makers, service providers and institutions must involve the public so that services and programs are accessible and appropriate to the people who are entitled to use them.

There are a series of principles, laid out such that we eliminate all poverty, eliminate all injustice, eliminate all discrimination and move towards paradise on earth in Ontario. Now, the Premier's Council material appears to be no longer interested in unsolicited innovation. They are certainly not interested in funding it. But they do want to eliminate poverty and hatred. It is a lovely statement of ideals, and I do not know if I am very cynical in saying that it seems to me absolutely unrealistic, and with Michael Decter's remark about Chou en Lai it seemed that it would fit very well in China or in Eastern Europe a few years ago, it is the sort of statement I saw from them. We are not talking about people being wealthy, we are just talking about equitable. If we could take away income from the top group of the population and make everyone the same, then the vision of social justice would be satisfied. I get a little alarmed when I look at what has happened in the collapse in Eastern Europe and I look at what has happened to their health-care system, which is what we claim we want to move towards. Yet when you look at China, when they had the rural economic reform, the first thing that they trashed was the entire rural health network. East Germany has a fairly good system, not that far from what we are trying to do. When they merged with the West, the first thing they did was to trash their system and they are trying to put in a West German type system.

Michael Decter noted that the *Canada Health Act* was comparatively narrow in its definition of what insured services were, and we are talking now about broad determinants of health. But I am never quite sure, when you operationalize that, what it means. Should we be paying for exercise classes? If I like reading and that will make me happy and enhance my well-being, do you pay for my books — well, I guess you do through public libraries. Now we are being reminded that medical care is not sufficient for health. So saying it is not sufficient does not mean that we can eliminate it. Technology sometimes may re-medicalize things and allow a technological "fix." I know the concept of the technological fix is not in vogue, but it is nonetheless sometimes true and let me give you a few examples. In the Soviet Union during the Tsarist period they had a terrible problem with typhoid fever, and they had humane physicians going out doing community development work to try and tell the peasants about improving their health, improving their lifestyles, and everything else to try and decrease the incidence of typhoid fever. Then a bunch of sanitary engineers came and put in sewage pipes, and — surprise! That did a better job of eliminating typhoid fever than all of the community development work by the physicians. The humanistic physicians fought the sanitary engineers because they saw it as a quick technological fix. They lost that battle. I will give you another example. In the days of the sabre tooth tiger, I would have been severely disabled. I would have stumbled off cliffs. Because I have a pair of glasses, I am not disabled. I do not need an aide, I do not need a homemaker. I would love a homemaker, but I do not need one, because with a pair of glasses I am no longer disabled. Someone mentioned before the fear that hip replacements or lens replacements would not be done for the elderly. Those are probably the most cost effective sorts of things to do, because you remove someone from dependency and allow them to function. As Maimonides said, "the highest form of charity is to help someone help themselves." I suspect that the advancements in micro-biology and genetic engineering will mean that in the not too distant future we will understand the biochemical bases of a lot of the serious mental illnesses, in which case schizophrenia may be very similar to what diabetes is now. Diabetics do not need an entire support system. They obviously have to watch their diets, and there are things that can precipitate crises. Certainly current treatment is not a total technological fix, but a diabetic who has proper medical management and the right support does not need to be in that much contact with the health-care system. It may be the same for a number of other conditions.

I think we have to be prepared to allow things to be re-medicalized, if what that may do is end some of this long-term dependency, and I think again we are a little too fixated on the current level of technological development and seeing all the technology as this horrible scary thing which is just going to keep people alive, when, "Why don't they die nicely and quietly?" However, I cannot quite reconcile that with our objection to smoking on cost-effectiveness grounds. Because smoking probably is the cheapest thing going. If you get lung cancer, it kills you off fast, just before you collect your pension which implies that maybe we should look at the benefit side, and not just as the costs. Anyway, I think what I am trying to say is that in the discussion of innovation, there may be a certain risk of throwing babies out with bath water. Mrs. Armit spoke about crossroads and the question of where we are going. I am reminded of the conversation between Alice and the Cheshire Cat, where Alice asks the Cat which way she should go. The Cat asks where she wants to go. Alice says she does not much care and the Cat says, well then it does not matter which way she goes. Now if we do care where we want to go, then I presumably hope and trust that we are going in the right direction. We cannot be quite as sanguine as Alice, and the remark I think I will conclude with in terms of challenges is the insight by Aaron Wildavsky, who is an American political scientist. What he says is that you never, ever, solve problems. What you do is you replace one set of problems with a different set of problems. The issue then is which set of problems you prefer. I think that given that sort of insight, which may make us feel a bit better, the set of problems we have in overall terms probably could be a lot worse.

INITIATIVES

One of the very successful additions to the Health Care: Innovation, Impact and Challenge conference was a large number of displays of health initiatives. Twenty-five exhibitors came and presented their current projects, including: research on Diabetes, the Canadian Medical Association, the Health Policy Research and Evaluation Unit at Queen's, the Community Registry of Nurses for Deep River & District, the Geriatric Assessment Program, Consumer Health Information Service, the Premier's Council on Health, Well-Being and Social Justice, and many others. Several of the demonstrators were able to give us a written report on their activities and we have included those in this report.

Computerized Nursing Care Plan Project

Phyllis Patterson, Tanya Magee, Janet Brophy, Gordon Tait, Mary Jo Haddad

Current emphasis on the provision of quality patient care and professional accountability necessitates the development of clinical tools which facilitate professional nursing practice. Although nurses recognize the value of planning care, many view writing care plans as time consuming paperwork mandated by professional nursing bodies, accreditation standards, and hospital policy. The purpose of the Computerized Nursing Care Plan Project is to develop computer software that will enable practitioners to create comprehensive, individualized, and clinically relevant plans of care in a time-efficient manner. The two-year project is funded by the Premier's Council on Health, Well-being, and Social Justice through the Health Innovation/Strategies Fund.

The task for the project team is to design original software using Macintosh computers with a "point-and-click" interface requiring minimal use of the keyboard, to develop a database of patient problems and nursing interventions, and to implement the system on four clinical units. This presentation provides an overview of the project team's experience in designing software and creating a database for use in the clinical setting at the Hospital for Sick Children, Toronto.

Phyllis Patterson, RN, BAA (Nursing), Tanya Magee, RN, BN; Janet Brophy, RN, BScN; Gordon Tait, PhD; Mary Jo Haddad, RN, BScN, at the Hospital for Sick Children, Toronto.

ASSESSMENT

Initial assessment of care-planning needs involved evaluating current policy and practice, reviewing the literature, surveying other paediatric institutions, and engaging in discussion with nurses in all areas of nursing practice. Evaluation of current practice showed that patient problems were not identified on 37 percent of the care plans and that the nurses did not perceive the current care plans to be helpful in organizing or directing patient care. Other Canadian paediatric hospitals indicated that care plans were or were soon to become part of the patient's permanent record. Standard care plans were used in the majority of institutions to act as a reference for the development of individualized care plans. The current trend was towards nursing diagnosis-focused care plans.

Basic assumptions on which the development of the computer-supported plans of care were based evolved in discussions with nurses. Nurses want the plan of care to be relevant for the child's age, developmental stage, and clinical condition; patient-specific, not "standard care"; problem-focused; supportive of family-centred care; flexible, and easy to revise and individualize.

DESIGN

User friendliness and system flexibility were primary goals in designing the software. Consistent screen design, a point-and-click interface requiring minimal use of the keyboard, and a logical progression through the process of developing a plan of care all contribute to user friendly software. Staff nurses provided input regarding program functions and screen design. Prototype software was tested in the clinical setting and revised based on user feedback. Issues of system integrity and patient confidentiality required consideration. To access the system the user was required "sign on" and enter a password. An audit trail documents all entries and changes to the plan of care.

Developing the database has involved identifying patient problems and interventions for the acutely ill paediatric patient population. The nurse selects patient-appropriate problems and interventions from scrolling lists. A consistent language to identify patient problems and an organizational framework is necessary for computerization. Nursing diagnoses developed by the North American Nursing Diagnosis Association (NANDA) have been used to identify patient problems. The diagnoses have been grouped according to a Systems framework and *Gordon's Functional Health Patterns*. The interventions reflect current clinical practice and research, and have been validated by practitioners and clinical experts.

IMPLEMENTATION

To date, the project team has designed and developed prototype software using HyperCard R; developed a database of 45 nursing diagnoses with over 2,500 accompanying interventions; and implemented the system in the Paediatric Intensive Care Unit (PICU) and the Cardiology/Cardiovascular Unit.

RESULTS

The project goals are to demonstrate an improvement in the quality of care plans and compliance with present policy, not to increase the time required to create a written plan of care; assess whether the use of computerized care plans contribute to continuity of care between units; and determine whether the use of computerized care plans influences job satisfaction and quality of work life.

The system has been implemented for two months on the clinical units. Daily statistics gathered over a four-week period one month after implementation demonstrate that the percentage of completed plans of care has increased from 63 percent to 84 percent in PICU. The average time required by project nurses to create a computer-supported Plan of Care (PPC) is 82 percent less than the time required to write a PPC. The average time for staff nurses to develop a computer-supported PPC is 12 minutes. The time needed to create a PPC on the computer is less than the estimated time of 15 minutes required to write a PPC.

CONCLUSIONS

The Computerized Nursing Care Plan Project is an exciting innovation that supports nursing in the provision of quality, professional care to the acutely ill paediatric patient.

The Consumer Health Information Service

Susan Murray and Joanne G. Marshall

In this paper, we will discuss the origin and background of Ontario's new Consumer Health Information Service located at the Metropolitan Toronto Reference Library and as well as the operation of the service and some of our experiences to date.

ORIGIN AND BACKGROUND

The Consumer Health Information Service (CHIS) is a pilot project supported by the Health Strategies Fund of the Premier's Council on Health, Well-being and Social Justice. Our mission is to improve access to health information for Ontario citizens by:

- creating a reliable and up-to-date collection of consumer health materials in print and electronic form,

- providing the means for consumers to become more informed about their health,

- facilitating the use of specialized health information sources through referrals, and

---

Susan Murray, Coordinator Consumer Health Information Service, Metropolitan Toronto Reference Library and Joanne Marshall, Associate Professor, Faculty of Library and Information Science, University of Toronto, and Chairperson, Management Committee, Consumer Health Information Service.

- supporting the provision of health information in public libraries across the province.

The project was initiated by the Consumers' Association of Canada (CAC), Ontario. In its policy statement (1989), the Association stated that health-care consumers have the right to be informed; the right to be respected as an individual with a major responsibility for his or her own health care; and the right to participate in health-care decision making. Members of the CAC (Ontario) Health Committee asked Professor Joanne Marshall of the University of Toronto Faculty of Library and Information Science to develop a proposal for the service and its evaluation. This partnership soon grew to include the Metropolitan Toronto Reference Library, The Toronto Hospital and the Centre for Health Promotion at the University of Toronto.

At another level of partnership, CHIS can be seen as an innovative and dynamic partnership between the Premier's Council on Health, Well-being and Social Justice, which has provided the funding for CHIS, and the Ministry of Culture and Communications, which funds the public libraries in the province.

The Consumers' Association is not alone in its concern about the informed health-care consumer. Ontario government reports such as *Health for All Ontario* (1987), *Toward a Shared Direction for Health* (1987), and *From Vision to Action* (1989) have all supported increased public participation in health care, both at the level of consumer decision making and health policy.

The World Health Organization has set a goal of "Health for All by the Year 2000" and we believe that libraries and librarians have an important part to play in ensuring that this goal includes "Health Information for All." Consumers require access to information to make informed decisions about their own health, that of their family members and friends and to participate in health policy and planning discussions at the community level. Only by knowing the pros and cons of a treatment, a drug, a lifestyle change or even a health-care delivery innovation such as the smart card, can consumers make effective and responsible choices. CHIS provides a way for consumers to access the information they need in such situations.

Many of the problems experienced by consumers in obtaining health information are problems of accessibility rather than availability, i.e., a great deal of health information is being created by commercial publishers, government and voluntary health organizations, but it has been very difficult for consumers to find out about these sources, locate them and evaluate their content. Traditionally, hospital and medical school libraries have served health-care providers rather than consumers, and opportunities for developing an expanded consumer service role in the current fiscal situation are extremely limited. Public libraries are responsive to the consumer movement, but in the past they have also been wary about infringing on the knowledge domains of powerful professions such as medicine and law.

CHIS is the first major, funded provincial service dedicated exclusively to the collection and dissemination of consumer health information. As such, it has the potential to serve as a focal library and a provincial health information resource for consumers who have access to 1,500 library locations across the province. CHIS can support the provision of health information in libraries across Ontario by developing resource guides and lists of recommended materials for collections, by offering educational opportunities for library staff and by continuing to be available as an in-depth collection and source of expertise.

The CHIS model is in keeping with the *Ontario Public Library Strategic Plan* (1990) and the vision of a provincial public library-based information network. We are very excited about CHIS's potential to meet the goals of the public library strategic plan while at the same time assisting the Ministry of Health to attain its goal of enabling informed choice by health-care consumers.

OPERATION AND EXPERIENCE TO DATE

The CHIS proposal was funded by the Premier's Council in the fall of 1991. The proposal for the Consumer Health Information Service was based on two needs assessments designed by Professor Marshall. During 1990-91 a questionnaire was sent to members of the CAC (Ontario) Consumer Panel to explore consumers' experiences in obtaining health information. A second survey funded by the Ministry of Culture and Communications studied the provision of health information in Ontario public libraries.

The coordinator and assistant coordinator were hired in January 1992 and service to the public began in mid-February. The service has a staff of five: two full-time librarians (the coordinator and assistant coordinator), a part-time librarian, a part-time library technician located at The Toronto Hospital and a part-time clerical assistant. A 1-800 telephone service covering the province began in April 1992. The project will continue in its current form until March 1993, after which we hope that continuing sources of funding will be found.

Free and confidential reference service is provided by experienced health librarians for 24 hours a week. The CHIS collection is available for use at other times that the library is open, but CHIS staff members are not available to provide assistance. Residents in the Toronto area are encouraged to visit CHIS and use the collection directly. Materials cannot be borrowed, but a photocopy machine is available. Information packages can be prepared for mailing or picked up in the library. The 1-800 number is staffed for 20 hours a week.

The project is governed by a Management Committee consisting of representatives of the five partners. An Advisory Committee, consisting of consumers, health professionals and others with expertise related to the project provides advice on the development of the service and assists in reviewing materials for the collection. The committee has also agreed to help us in developing strategies for future funding.

Each of the five partners in the project plays an important role. CAC (Ontario) ensures that the service is consumer-driven by providing direct input into the development and marketing of the service. The Faculty of Library and Information Science at the University of Toronto has guided the development of the service and is responsible for the evaluation component. The Metropolitan Toronto Reference Library is the host site and financial administrator of the project. A part-time library technician located at The Fudger Library of The Toronto Hospital is a key member of the staff who provides access to the professional health sciences literature when it is required. Health-care providers at the hospital also serve on the Advisory Committee. Participation by the Centre for Health Promotion at the University of Toronto ensures that wellness — as well as illness — information is emphasized.

On a day-to-day basis, information is provided at CHIS through:

- an up-to-date collection of consumer health books, pamphlets, magazines, newsletters and professional journals (approximately 500 books and 110 journal titles by the end of the project);

- computer databases, including *Health Reference Center, MDX Health Digest*, and *Patient Drug Information*;

- files on specific health topics containing a variety of materials such as newspaper and magazine articles, pamphlets, book lists, etc;

- brief resource guides on specific health topics are being developed which will be particularly useful to consumers who are unable to make an in-person visit;

- reviews of consumer health materials from authoritative sources including published reviews and reviews prepared for CHIS by health-care providers and consumers;

- lists of consumer health books, magazines and other materials that would be helpful to public libraries, health libraries, health agencies and health-care providers in Ontario (e.g., a guide to Canadian consumer health sources);

- access to other specialized collections through CHIS, e.g., CHIS can link into the network of health science libraries via The Toronto Hospital; and

- suggestions of other self-help groups, community and provincial health organizations and agencies, etc.

CHIS provides information on a variety of topics including the determinants of health, health promotion, prevention, wellness, drugs, and diseases such as Crohn's disease, diabetes, epilepsy, etc. Information on a range of therapies including medicine, chiropractic, acupuncture, homeopathy, massage therapy, etc. is also available. With the new regulated health professions legislation pending, CHIS also has information available on the training, education and qualifications of the various professions,

Detailed records are kept of CHIS enquiries and users are asked to complete a brief feedback form about the service. If users indicate that they used (or might use) the information to make a health decision, they are asked if they would be willing to be contacted again. These users are asked to provide a more detailed information case study indicating the situation that led them to make a request from CHIS, what information they received and how they used the information. Respondents names are kept confidential and only seen by CHIS staff members and evaluators.

As of June 1992, CHIS had received 1,164 walk-in inquiries and 1,590 requests by telephone. More than 30 percent of these inquiries resulted in either the preparation of information packages or the provision of in-depth service by CHIS staff. Our most popular topics currently are women's health issues, drugs, health promotion, depression, chronic fatigue and prostatic diseases. The most frequent user is a female between 30 and 40 years of age. We have found that, in many cases, women are requesting information for other family members or friends.

Comments from consumers have been extremely positive. A number of individuals have said that they used information provided by CHIS to make a health-care or lifestyle decision. To quote one questionnaire:

> I was very impressed with the concept behind the service and the way the service was carried out. I never expected to ask a question over the phone and be sent numerous articles addressing exactly the questions I wanted answered. Your database appears quite extensive. Having had experience with library research techniques, I know how much searching is necessary to find the perfect sources of information. For people without these skills the information would never get to them. In the area of health and medicine it is extremely important to be an educated consumer; you are making it possible for people to get all the facts about issues so crucial to their lives. The service is invaluable.

The CHIS pilot project ends in March 1993 and we are actively seeking funding to continue the service.

References

Acknowledgements: The Consumer Health Information Service is a team effort of the Staff (Susan Murray, Sharon Taylor, Marietta Forster Haberer, Stan Fettes and Cathy Pak); the Management Committee (Joanne Marshall, Sue Beck, Lucienne Bushnell, Frances Schwenger, Jennifer Bayne and Peggy Schultz); and the Advisory Committee (Mary Breen, Wendy Campbell, David Caspari, June Engel, Fred Fallis, Verla Fortier, Paul Gamble, Gordon Hardacre, Anne Louis Heron, Cathy Paul, Melanie Rantucci, Rose Rubino and Jackie Smith). We would also like to acknowledge the assistance of Linda Diener, the Metropolitan Toronto Reference Library staff and students from the University of Toronto and Seneca College.

Ontario, Health Care System Committee *From Vision to Action: Report* (Toronto: Premier's Council on Health Strategy, 1989)

Ontario, Panel on Health Goals for Ontario. *Health for all Ontario: Report* (Toronto: Ontario Ministry of Health, 1987)

Marshall J.G., C. Sewards and E. Dilworth "Health information services in Ontario public libraries," *Canadian Library Journal* (48, 1 (1991):37-44.

Ontario, Ontario Ministry of Culture and Communications and Ontario Library Association, *Ontario Public Library Strategic Plan: One Place to Look 1990.*

Consumers' Association of Canada, *Policy Statement on Consumers and Health Care* (Ottawa, 1989).

Ontario, Ontario Health Review Panel, *Toward a Shared Direction for Health in Ontario* (Toronto: Ontario Ministry of Health, 1987).

Nursing Needs in the Nineties: Results of a Feasibility Study Prepared for the Ministry of Health

Leslie Martel and Judy Coleman

ABSTRACT

In September 1991 the Community Registry of Nurses for Deep River &
District received a grant from the Ministry of Health to undertake a market
survey. This study focused on the nursing needs and preferences of the general
public and whether there were sufficient nurses to form a Registry and how it
would fit in with existing services. This paper presents some of the highlights
from this study.

INTRODUCTION

Deep River is a small town on the Ottawa River 200 Kms. west of Ottawa. The
population of Deep River is approximately 4,200 and there are an additional
3,000 people from the surrounding townships. Deep River is the bedroom
community for the scientific establishment of Chalk River Nuclear Laboratories. The main objective of this market study was to evaluate the current need
for a Nursing Registry in Deep River that would provide the best possible
nursing care to patients in their home on a 24 hour basis. A second objective

Leslie Martel, RN and Judy Coleman, RN, Community Registry of Nurses for Deep
River & District.

was to examine the attitudes of the local nurses as well as the larger scale health-care providers (e.g., hospital and Home Care) in the community towards the establishment of such a Nursing Registry.

SURVEY OF THE GENERAL PUBLIC

David Prentice of Design House, a market research company in Pembroke, was hired to coordinate the survey. In October of 1991, 300 non-business addresses were chosen at random from the local phone book and sent a survey form. A total of 111 completed forms were returned for tabulation and analysis by 11 December 1991, for a response rate of 37 percent. While this is a reasonable return rate to have expected, there is an obvious self-selection bias that is built into such a survey. Due to the nature of the survey regarding long-term health-care options, respondents tended to be older and from smaller households than the population as a whole. (See Table 1.) A summary of the demographics of the respondents versus those of the total population can be seen here. The results tend to show a high level of support from the segment of the population most likely to need it. As the younger people continue to leave small towns like Deep River for larger urban centres, the percentage of "older" people will continue to grow.

Respondents were asked to rank their preference for continuing care, and the majority by far (77 percent) chose in-home care, followed by hospital (10 percent) and Nursing Home (5 percent). Respondents were asked to indicate their level of agreement with various situations. Some 68 percent agreed with the statement that, "If a loved one were dying and requested that he/she be allowed to die at home, I would support that decision provided that there is a suitable support system available."

The person requiring such health care tends in the majority (68 percent) to be a senior citizen, with the rest evenly split between disabled (27 percent) and terminally ill (23 percent). Upon further examination of the data, the consultant developed another tabulation that determined that 41 percent of the total sample (see Table 2) have either a current need for nursing care or a "likely" need in the future.

This rather large number is consistent with the forecast that the need for such care will greatly increase. Incidence is somewhat higher among older respondents and those with lower incomes and a secondary education or less. Three-quarters of the 41 percent also preferred in-home care over hospital or nursing homes for long-term nursing care. Nearly 23 percent of the respondents foresee a need for respite care service within the next five to ten years.

Table 1. *Deep River Demographics Versus Survey Sample*

	Total Survey	Deep River K0J 1P0
Population (1986)		4,602
Tax Filers (1988)		3,350
Households (1986)		1,670
Sample (1991)	111	74
% of Sample	100%	67%
ADULT AGE		
<45	15%	50%
45 – 64	43%	34%
65 +	43%	17%
HOUSEHOLD SIZE		
1 person	22%	19%
2 persons	51%	34%
3 persons	13%	15%
4 or 5 persons	15%	29%
6+ persons	1%	2%
Average	2	3
INCOME	(HOUSEHOLD)	(HOUSEHOLD)
<20,000	12%	
$20,000 – $35,000	22%	
$35,000 – $50,000	21%	
> $50,000	45%	
Median	$35,000-$50,000	$48,746
		INDIVIDUAL
<15,000		37%
$15,000 – $25,000		14%
$25,000 – $35,000		16%
$35,000 – $50,000		17%
>$50,000		16%
Median		$24,300
Index vs. Ontario		126
Tax Filers per Household		2

Surveys requested Postal Codes; the Deep River code was only one for which there was a statistically reliable number of questionnaire returns.
Survey % is adjusted for non-response.
Median Household Income calculated by Quire Market Information, Mississauga.

Source: Statistics Canada, 1988.

Table 2. *Community Registry: Residents, Need Nursing Care Now/In Future*

All Respondents

| | | Age | | | Education | |
| | Total | Under 45 to 65 | | | Primy/ | Post- |
	Total	45	64	Plus	Secndy	Secndy
UNWEIGHTED BASE	111	15	45	45	45	54
		14%	41%	41%	41%	49%
Yes/Likely	45	6	16	21	23	18
	41%	40%	36%	47%	51%	33%
NO RESPONSE	66	9	29	24	22	36
	59%	60%	64%	53%	49%	67%
Chi Square	0.00	0.00				
	p=.999	p=.999				

Source: Statistics Canada.

Chart 1. *The General Public's Preferences for Nursing Care Options*

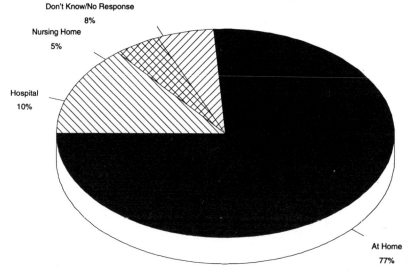

Don't Know/No Response
8%

Nursing Home
5%

Hospital
10%

At Home
77%

Source: Authors' compilation.

Although there is a large percentage (84 percent) enrolled in a private health care insurance plan, 45 percent of respondents did not know the extent of their insurance coverage. Thus the positive response was not unduly influenced by this factor.

NURSES

A second survey was conducted among nurses in the area to assess their current employment and their interest in the Registry. Questionnaires were sent out to 90 nurses and 49 were returned. Of the respondents 20 percent were employed full-time, 49 percent were part-time and 24 percent were not employed in nursing at all. There were 35 percent of the respondents that were very interested in joining the Registry (Chart 2). Interest tended to be among those who were less than fully employed. This indicates that the Registry would promote fuller employment of nurses without hurting existing full-time em-ployed nurses, since only one full-time nurse indicated "some interest" in joining a Registry.

Chart 2. *Nurses Interested in Joining a Registry*

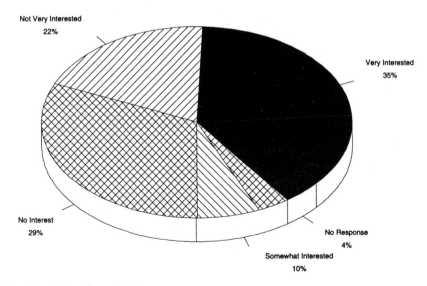

Source: Authors' compilation.

DOCTORS AND HEALTH PROFESSIONALS

A total of 25 interviews were conducted with doctors and other health-care professionals in Deep River and Pembroke. Although there was not a statistically valid number of respondents for quantitative analysis, there was a clear indication that the health professionals who were consulted, considered the Community Registry of Nurses for Deep River and District to be a good idea. All local doctors expressed a willingness to make home visits to their patients as required. Several of the doctors wrote or promised to write letters of endorsement which are included in the study. When asked how the Registry would fit into the existing services for Deep River and Area residents, most respondents tended to feel that the Registry would fit in well. Some mentioned that it offered another choice, that it would fit well between Home Care and the hospital or complement existing services.

CONCLUSION

The results of the survey of all people concerned with the establishment of a Nursing Registry in Deep River indicated a positive response from all segments. In the 1991 Ministry of Health's publication *Redirection of Long-Term Care and Support Services in Ontario*, A Public Consultation Paper, there is a move towards providing more care in the home. Our survey indicates that there is strong public support in Deep River for this move. The Registry of Nurses will be there as a support service to help make this a reality.

Uniform Clinical Data Set
A Comprehensive Clinical
Information System

Wilma M. Hopman

The Uniform Clinical Data Set (UCDS) is an innovative computer screening system that has many applications both in the Canadian and the American health-care systems. It is designed to gather data in a systematic and consistent manner, and has two primary uses. The first is to collect data critical for the measurement and uniform evaluation of the quality and medical necessity of care received by patients during hospitalization. The second is to develop detailed databases for epidemiological research.

The UCDS was developed through the collaborative efforts of the Health Care Financing Administration (the U.S. federal agency that controls funding for the Medicare and Medicaid programs), several Peer Review Organizations (state-based agencies designed to monitor utilization and quality for Medicare and Medicaid beneficiaries) and clinical researchers from several academic centres including Case Mix Research at Queen's University and the Boston University Medical Center.

The impetus for its development was to provide the Peer Review Organizations with a mechanism for screening in-patient cases for utilization and quality. Currently, nurses evaluate the medical record and refer it to a physician if they determine that a potential problem exists. Although they have specific guidelines to follow, the process remains somewhat subjective, and there is wide variation in referral rates across the Peer Review Organizations.

Wilma M. Hopman, BA, MA, Case Mix Research, Department of Community Health and Epidemiology, Queen's University, Kingston.

Under UCDS review procedures, trained medical abstractors enter data from the chart into collection screens. The abstractor needs no knowledge of computers in order to use the system. All utilities such as formatting disks, backing up data onto diskettes, and deleting old cases are menu options in the UCDS primary menu, and are discussed during the abstractor training. To enter the data collection screens, the reviewer selects the first option from the primary menu, and selects the case he or she wishes to review.

Close to 1,800 data elements exist in the UCDS, including risk factors such as severity of illness, comorbid conditions, history and physical findings and laboratory values, treatment processes such as results of diagnostic tests, operative episodes and hospital course, and outcomes such as discharge status and planning. The average in-patient chart contains approximately 300 of these data elements. They are contained in a series of 17 screens, as outlined, with examples, below.

THE DATA COLLECTION SCREENS

Screen Q   *Administrative Information*: patient identification code and date of birth, admission and discharge date, diagnosis and procedure codes, discharge disposition.

Screen A   *Sociodemographic Data*: admission path, caregiver, patient race, occupational status, insurance source, current ambulatory care.

Screen B   *Admission Status*: activities of daily living prior to admission, height, weight, vital signs.

Screen C   *Admission Medication History:* current medications at admission, history of alcohol or tobacco use, drug/dye allergy or poisoning, radiation exposure, medications administered in emergency room.

Screen D   *History of Permanent Anatomic Changes*: major organ removal, replaced body parts (pacemaker, cardiac valves, hip, etc.) amputation of major limb, organ transplant.

Screen E   *History and Physical 1*: chronic or current neurological, cardiac, pulmonary and psychiatric disease, history of neurological, vascular or pulmonary surgery, cancer.

Screen F   *History and Physical 2*: chronic gastrointestinal, hepatobili-
                  ary, pancreatic, endocrine and autoimmune disease, history
                  of gastrointestinal or endocrine surgery, current gastrointes-
                  tinal findings, HIV+.

Screen G   *History and Physical 3*: chronic or current urologic or obstet-
                  rical/gynecological disease, musculoskeletal and cutaneous
                  exam findings, current neonate findings.

Screen H   *Laboratory Findings*: chemistry, hematology, urinalysis,
                  blood gases, microbiology, cytology/histology.

Screen I   *Diagnostic Tests 1*: chest x-ray, upper GI, barium
                  enema/swallow, gallbladder, bone/spinal x-ray, CT scan,
                  MRI, KUB/abdominal, IVP/urogram, nuclear medicine iso-
                  topic studies, ultrasound.

Screen J   *Diagnostic Tests 2*: EKG, cardiac catheterization, ventricu-
                  logram, arteriogram, angiogram, EEG, GI motility,
                  echocardiogram, pulmonary function.

Screen K   *Endoscopic Procedures*: arthroscopy, cystoscopy/ cysto-
                  gram, laparoscopy, hysteroscopy, bronchoscopy/ laryngos-
                  copy, upper GI endoscopy, ERCP.

Screen L   *Operative Episodes*: operative procedures done during the
                  hospitalization, date of operation, anaesthetic type, anaes-
                  thetic risk, vascular access lines, surgical wound classifica-
                  tion, adverse intra-operative occurrences, tissue findings.

Screen M   *Treatment Interventions*: blood products, inhalation therapy,
                  professional services, prescribed medications, delivery sys-
                  tems for and adverse reactions to medications.

Screen N   *Hospital Course*: special care unit episodes, do not resusci-
                  tate order and date, adverse occurrences, trauma suffered in
                  hospital, infections, prolonged stay.

Screen O   *Discharge Status*: discharge vital signs, discharge physical
                  exam findings, discharge x-rays.

Screen P   *Discharge Planning*: discharge activities of daily living, care giver, follow-up plans, therapies, medications, discharge diagnoses and disposition.

THE DATA COLLECTION GUIDELINES

The abstractors follow a series of guidelines relating to various aspects of the data collection process. For example, for each individual data element, the most likely location(s) in the medical record are cited in the UCDS data collection manual. For some data elements with multiple sources, an order of preference is given. For example, for history and physical screens, medical student notes are not used unless no other source of data is available and the notes are countersigned by the attending physician. Also, the discharge summary is excluded as the source of data for elements that are collected to assess the patient's condition at admission, since the discharge summary reflects the patient's condition after treatment.

The reviewers are also given synonymous words and phrases to aid in identifying each data element. For example, under current cardiovascular exam findings, the presence of pulmonary edema is a collected data element. Abstractors are instructed to look for such key words as pulmonary effusion, wet lungs, or frothy sputum in evaluating this element. Similarly, under current pulmonary findings, to determine the presence of laboured breathing, abstractors are directed to look for key words such as dyspnea, laboured breathing, fighting for air, or S.O.B.

To facilitate the accurate collection of medications, the UCDS data collection software contains a drug reference list. As a medication is typed in, the portion of the list that corresponds alphabetically to the typed name will appear. The abstractor can than select the appropriate name from the list and automatically enter the correct drug. The reviewer is warned with a beep if he or she attempts to enter a drug name that is not contained in the list. The system will accept these drugs, however, since certain experimental drugs are not yet on the list.

Finally, the reviewers are given certain rules or data collection principles, which they follow to collect measurements that change over time and in determining abnormal values. For example, a number of data elements are collected with reference to specific periods of the hospital stay. In general, data describing the condition of the patient at admission are those collected within the first 24 hours of the stay, although for certain lab tests such as cardiac enzymes the window is within 48 hours of admission.

If more that one finding was recorded in the relevant interval, the more abnormal value is collected. In the case of vital signs, the highest and lowest recorded values are collected. In the case of the more complex diagnostic tests such as endoscopy and radiology, abnormal findings from all tests are recorded. For some labs, the most abnormal ("worst") result obtained in the interval between the first 24 hours and the last reported value is also collected. In all instances, the dates of performance of the test are collected. In collecting the data that describes patient status at discharge, the physical examination results and the vital signs must have been obtained within 24 hours of discharge.

THE DECISION-MAKING ALGORITHMS

Once the data is collected, it is processed through clinical decision rules, or algorithms, which identify cases requiring additional review. An algorithm is defined as a set of rules or systematic method for solving problems or reaching decisions. In the UCDS, the algorithms use the data abstracted from the medical record to "decide" whether or not a case should be sent to a physician for utilization or quality of care review.

The UCDS algorithms consist of a body of several thousand rules generated by expert consensus panels. These rules are grouped into modules, three of which evaluate the appropriateness of admission, one of which contains the generic quality screening rules, and one of which evaluates the discharge planning. The three appropriateness-of-admission (or utilization) modules consist of elective surgery algorithms; which evaluate the common and important surgical admissions; the disease specific algorithms, which evaluate major types of medical conditions such as diabetes and lung cancer; and the organ system module, evaluating conditions such as renal failure and anemia.

Generic quality modules are more specific and are based on the six quality screens as outlined by HCFA. The first of these consists of a number of rules dealing with adequacy of discharge planning. The second evaluates patient stability at discharge, particularly temperature, pulse, blood pressure and intravenous medications in the 24 hours prior to discharge. It also looks for any abnormal results not addressed during the hospitalization. The third quality screen deals with death during or after elective surgery, in special care units, or any unexplained death. The fourth deals with nosocomial infections, and the fifth evaluates unplanned returns to surgery. The sixth quality screen has many components, and deals with iatrogenic events such as drug reactions, fall with injury, life-threatening anesthesia complication or transfusion error, hospital-acquired decubitus ulcers and other care resulting in life-threatening complications.

The discharge modules are based on the same information as the first of the generic quality screens (adequacy of discharge planning), but go into much greater detail. These rules evaluate discharge vital signs and physical examination data, along with discharge activities of daily living, therapies and follow-up plans.

These case-finding algorithms are extensive, and cover many potential problems with utilization or quality of care. They are, however, not exhaustive, and the nurse reviewers are given the option to refer to a physician peer reviewer if they detect a quality or utilization problem not accounted for by the algorithms.

CONCLUSIONS

The UCDS has improved the ability of Peer Review Organizations and individual health-care providers to identify those patients that have received substandard care. The UCDS data can also be linked to a broad base of utilization and demographic data and provider characteristics, which can be used to assess the effectiveness of different approaches to treating a medical problem.

The Health Care Financing Administration is planning to implement the UCDS nationwide. Case Mix Research at Queen's University has been involved in the pilot and field testing of the software, evaluation of preliminary data, training in the use of the software, and technical support. Current work includes continued software training and support, evaluation and analysis of 20,000 abstracted charts from six Peer Review Organizations, and continued updating and revisions of the clinical algorithms.

Additional current work includes the Elective Surgery Algorithm Project, a collaborative effort with Case Mix Research, Boston University and several Peer Review Organizations, funded by the Health Care Financing Administration. Six high-cost and/or high-volume elective surgical procedures commonly performed on the Medicare population have been targeted for this study, which involves developing methodology for designing algorithms that are highly reflective of scientific knowledge and readily revised as the knowledge base changes. The algorithms developed for the six procedures will be programmed into the UCDS knowledge base. The methodology will be the basis for future algorithm design, for both surgical procedures and medical treatment.

Additional future work includes continuous updating of the clinical algorithms that already exist in the UCDS, as practice patterns change over time with the advent of new technologies. New algorithms will also be developed as the need arises. In addition, there will be changes to the software to accommodate the needs and interests of certain groups, such as individual hospitals that are interested only in the information associated with certain conditions rather than the entire database.

The UCDS is therefore a valuable tool with the potential to help providers evaluate and strengthen their internal quality assurance programs, as well as allowing providers, epidemiologists and other clinical researchers to use outcomes analysis and risk adjustment to identify the most effective methods of patient care.

Diabetes Education Manual: Survival Skills

R. Barrett, C. Bird, R. Houlden, and L. Revell

In order to meet the basic, educational needs of patients admitted to hospital with newly-diagnosed diabetes, we developed a Diabetes Education Manual to be used to establish consistency in patient teaching by nursing staff, medical staff and dietitians. Patients are instructed on "survival skills" to enable them to cope safely with their disease after leaving hospital. Seven colour-coded modules cover the following topics: what is diabetes, insulin, oral hypoglycaemic agents, the diabetic way of eating, hypoglycaemia, hyperglycaemia and sick day rules, and monitoring. The information is presented through a series of repeating, self-explanatory, coloured drawings and text written at a Grade 6-8 level. Laminated copies of the Manual are available on each nursing unit with measurable objectives for each module to direct the teaching, and assess the patients' learning. Non-laminated copies are given to patients to take home as reference manuals, with individualized notations having been made by any teaching team member.

Endocrinology Department, Kingston General Hospital, Kingston.

Children at Risk Programme: Staying-on-Track

Jane LaPalme

EARLY TRACKING, IDENTIFICATION AND REFERRAL SYSTEM FOR INFANTS AND YOUNG CHILDREN

In November 1989, the Leeds, Grenville and Lanark Health Unit and Beechgrove Children's Centre received a grant from the Health Innovation Fund of the Ontario Premier's Council on Health Strategy, for a three-and-a-half year period, in order to establish an early identification, tracking and referral system for young children in Brockville, Ontario. Brockville is a city of 20,000 in the rural community of Leeds, Grenville counties.

The goal of the funded project was to promote the healthy development of all children and their families. "Staying on Track" commenced operation in early 1990 with six principle objectives:

1. To set-up a community-wide early identification and tracking system in Brockville, Ontario which has the potential to track and assess *all* babies born in the area from one month to school entry at five-and-half years of age. As well, the intent is that the system will be transferable to other areas in Ontario with adaptations according to the unique characteristics of the community.

2. To evaluate the sensitivity and specificity of a number of question-naires, tests and observational scales and to evaluate their ability as indicators of child developmental functioning; social competence; and self-regulatory behaviour.

3.   To establish a database, and using multivariate statistical analysis, to examine the comparative contribution of a number of variables to developmental outcome of the child at five-and-a-half years of age. The data being collected broadens the usual focus of early screening systems to include sociodemographic characteristics; interaction between parents and child; parental attitudes and functioning; and child variables.

4.   Because long-term funding was not available to carry out longitudinal research, evaluation of the effectiveness of the intervention components of the tracking system on eventual outcome is being assessed utilizing a cohort design which allows time-lagged contrasts between age equivalent groups.

There are three cohorts:

1. Newborn Cohort:
This group was recruited in prenatal classes and through baby visits offered by the Public Health Nurses.
These infants are assessed at:
- one month
- six months
- eighteen months

2. Eighteen Month Cohort:
This group was recruited by phone. Old records were used to find children who were of the appropriate age. This group has never had any services provided previously in this community.
These children are assessed at:
- eighteen months
- two-and-a-half years
- three-and-a-half years

3. Preschool Cohort:
This group was recruited as they entered Junior Kindergarten. The Health Unit has always provided screening for this age group and they were offered the option of participating in the project.
These children are assessed at:
- three-and-a-half years
- four-and-a-half years
- five-and-a-half years

5. To provide child development and parenting information along with counselling as part of the data collection and assessment process. In addition, when children and families are identified with greater than normal needs or with developmental problems and are seen at risk for falling short of their potential; to carry out follow-up visits and where necessary, to make referrals to other agencies in the area.

6. To increase the cooperation and coordination of service provision for the young children and families in the area and particularly for the children identified by the tracking system as needing additional intervention. This process is facilitated by the "Staying On Track" Community Advisory Board, whose members represent the service agencies and various disciplines providing intervention services for young children and their families in the Brockville area.

Managing With Values:
The Road to Quality Management

Lynda Trommelen

INTRODUCTION

The challenge faced by hospital administrators in the 1990s is to maintain high quality patient care with the increasingly limited resources available. Collaboration, productivity improvement, refocusing of services and managing for value are big factors in the renewal process.

Staff costs represent 60 percent or more of hospital budgets. It is particularly important to ensure that the potential of this important resource is managed as effectively as possible. Staff morale has a major impact on the care patients receive. This in turn may affect recovery rates and length of stay. Staff satisfaction also has an impact on productivity, absenteeism rates, staff recruitment and retention.

However, the importance of employee involvement in the decision-making process in the workplace and the impact of employee satisfaction in organizational effectiveness, are often overlooked in the management of health-care personnel.

Employee participation in the decision-making process and the conditions of their work, plus a clear recognition of their contribution to the overall success of an organization, are key factors in positive communication in the unionized environment that exists in most hospitals.[1] Eleanor Caplan, Ontario's former Minister of Health, attempted to address this issue in the nurses in key decision-making committees within hospitals.[2] Other professional groups are now also interested in the same consideration.[3] An "ideal" hospital environment would be one in which all groups mutually

---

Lynda Trommelen, Director, Educational Services, Hotel Dieu Hospital, Kingston.

respected each other and supported the best efforts to serve the patients' needs. Competition for scarce resources fosters rivalry and inhibits cooperation. Clinicians and department managers tenaciously hold on to what they have, in the fear that budget cuts may seriously impair their ability to function.

Hospital administrators often find themselves in the role of mediators as they attempt to allocate limited resources among these sectors to ensure the best possible patient care. The hierarchical organizational structure of most hospitals creates further divisional barriers and inhibits interdisciplinary approaches to patient care and problem solving.

GOAL

At Hotel Dieu Hospital, Kingston a program has been initiated based on a participatory management approach that:

- respects and values the contributions of individual staff members, regardless of their position within the organization;
- encourages interdisciplinary approaches to problem solving and decision making, through a participative management style;
- fosters mutual respect and understanding through awareness of individual strengths and the importance of collaboration to put forth the best effort; and
- includes all members of the hospital community in the information, communication flow and decision-making process.

The overall goal of the program is to ensure quality patient care, and organizational effectiveness in an organization that can adapt more easily to the continued process of change in our health-care system.

Specific Objectives include:

1. to assess if participative management/employee involvement improves staff satisfaction;
2. to determine if increased staff involvement reduces absenteeism/stress related illnesses/grievances;
3. to determine if this approach can improve cooperation and collaboration between the working groups within the hospital (i.e., physicians, nursing, professional services, support staff and administration) to further enhance patient care;

4. to determine if an improvement in interdisciplinary working relation-
    ships can minimize duplication of efforts and maximize resource allo-
    cation;
5. to determine if increased employee involvement/participation produces
    new, more innovative solutions to hospital problems; and
6. to determine if such an approach could be adapted and implemented in
    other hospital settings.

Steps in Program Development included:

1984   - Organizational Needs survey

1985/86   - Review of the Hospital's Mission Statement

1987   - Development of a booklet stating the Hospital's Values

1988   - Introduction of the Myers-Briggs Type Indicator (MBTI) at a
            Senior Management Retreat as a tool to help bring about organiza-
            tional change

1989   - Similar workshops offered to Middle Managers and staff
            - Semi-annual planning days initiated
            - First staff-initiated Action Groups form
            - Open Staff Meetings initiated on regular basis

1990   - Workshops continue on a monthly basis for all staff
            - Follow-up workshops are offered to those who have attended
            previously to introduce new skills and applications
            - Action Groups continue to form as new issues emerge, and disband
            as issues are resolved
            - QA Report indicates improvement in key areas

1991   - Workshops continue for staff and are opened when space is avail-
            able to participants from other organizations wishing to learn more
            about the process
            - Communication survey highlights staff growth and involvement
            despite downsizing efforts within the hospital

1992   - Suggestions proposed by staff as improvements are reported
            monthly with feedback on actions in the Hospital Newsletter
            - Kaizen applications based workshops continue at the department
            level

OBSERVED RESULTS

(A) QA Report of Program, January 1990 yielded a 40% survey response from managers and staff surveyed.

1. How effective do you feel that the program has been in achieving its overall goals?

    a) greater staff morale 86%
    b) greater awareness of other hospital departments 89%
    c) more effective communication
       i) between departments 90%
       ii) between managers/employees 79%
       iii) between peers 90%

2. Have you observed any changes during the past year in your work environment?

50% responded Positively Comments included:
- we are building an energetic, innovative hospital
- more positive working environment
- more willingness to tolerate differences
- asks us to be more responsible
- allows us to speak out constructively
- giant steps in advancing personal growth and integrating staff into a productive cohesive unit

31% reported No Change Comments included:
- positive environment already existed and is being maintained
- more people need to attend workshops to make this work in our department

4% felt Negatively Comments included:
- manager not committed to the program
- authoritarian management style still exists in our department
- "us" versus "them" attitude still prevails

(B) Follow-up Evaluations/Surveys

Increased Staff Involvement in Decision-Making Process (1991/92)
- through staff participation on internal committees and at Open Staff Meetings

Increase in New Initiatives (1991/92)
- staff-initiated action groups developed around timely issues, e.g.,
- "Waste Watchers"
- multiculturalism
- sexual abuse awareness
- secretarial support
- parking concerns

Communication survey (December 1991) indicated
- satisfaction with openness of methods and opportunity for input
- greater tolerance and understanding between staff and management
- initiation of a staff suggestion box with a monthly Newsletter column to
  provide update on all ideas submitted for consideration

NEXT STEPS IN THE PROCESS

At a recent conference in Toronto, Jim Clemmer, the keynote speaker on "Total
Quality Management" illustrated this concept using 3 rings:

Chart 1. *Next Steps in the Process*

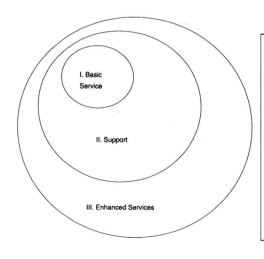

I. Basic Service

II. Support

III. Enhanced Services

I.   The first ring addressed the technical
     specifications and standards of
     Quality Assurance
     (i.e.: Hi-Tech – Clinical Care)

II. The second ring looks at how the
     systems and processes support the
     basic service.
     (i.e.: Administrative functions)

III. The third ring addresses the human
     dimension.
     (i.e.: Hi-Touch, sense of caring/
     personal treatment)

We have taken some major steps in achieving a culture that values quality of health care in a supportive work environment (outer ring). Our Departmental Quality Assurance indicators continue to assess performance at the inner ring level.

The hospital is currently re-organizing to provide a better framework for organizational effectiveness. This second level, the administrative support structure, will be our major focus in the immediate future. The traditional structure of hospitals no longer fits the current changes that require multidisciplinary approaches and greater functional accountability. Developing a more flexible and collaborative framework that responds more quickly and effectively is the next challenge.

Notes

[1] Edwin L. Stringer, Q.C., "Positive Communications in a Unionized Environment," *The Human Resource*, (Aug/Sept. 1988): 10-13. J. Trypuc, D. Abbey-Livingston, "Valued Workplaces: Hospital Snapshots," Publication #185 (The Ontario Hospital Association, 1991).

[2] Elinor Caplan, "Amendments to Ontario Regulation 518/88," statement presented at Queen's Park, Toronto, 15 February 1989.

[3] Allan McKeown, "Ontario's Nurses Seek Change in Health Care." OSMT Update, 5, 3 (May 1989): 24-25.

ACRONYMS

ACIP: Ambulatory Care Incentive Payment
AMA: American Medical Association
CAC: Consumers' Association of Canada
CCHFA: Canadian Council on Health-Care Facilities Accreditation
CCOTA: Coordinating Office on Health Technology Assessment
CGP: Confederation of General Practitioners
CHA: Canada Health Act
CHC: Community Health Centre
CHD: Coronary Heart Disease
CHIS: Consumer Health Information Service
CHO: Comprehensive Health Organization
CMA: Canadian Medical Association
CMG: Case Mix Group
COMSOC: Ministry of Community and Social Services
CPHA: Canadian Public Health Association
CPI: Consumer Price Index
CPP: Canada Pension Plan
CQI: Continuous Quality Improvement
CUPE: Canadian Union of Public Employees
DHC: District Health Council
DPA: Drugless Practitioners Act
DRG: Diagnosis Related Group
EPF: Established Programs Financing
HDA: Health Disciplines Act
HMO: Health Maintenance Organization
HMRI: Hospital Medical Records Institute
HPLR: Health Professions Legislation Review
HRA: Health Records Analyst
HRT: Health Records Technician
HSO: Health Service Organization
ICD: International Classification of Diseases
IPA: Independent Practice Association
MOH: Ministry of Health
OHA: Ontario Hospital Association
OAS: Old Age Security

OECD: Organisation for Economic Cooperation and Development
OHIP: Ontario Health Insurance Program
OMA: Ontario Medical Association
ONA: Ontario Nurses Association
PIN: Personal Identification Number
PPO: Preferred Provider Organization
PRO: Peer Review Organization
PROS: Plan Regional d'organisation de Service
PSI: Physicians Services Incorporated
PSRO: Professional Standards Review Organization
QA: Quality Assurance
RIW: Resource Intensity Weight
STATS CAN: Statistics Canada
UCDS: Uniform Clinical Data Set
WCB: Workers' Compensation Board
WHO: World Health Organization

Contributors

Amelita A. Armit is Assistant Deputy Minister, Health Services and Promotions Branch, Health and Welfare Canada. She has lectured in public administration, policy analysis and program evaluation. Her current responsibilities include health insurance and promotion and the National Health Research and Development Program.

Lynn Curry is a principal in Curry Adams & Associates of Ottawa. She has published an extensive series of papers, book chapters and monographs in the areas of general and professional education, program planning, design and evaluation.

Raisa Deber is Professor in the Department of Health Administration at the University of Toronto. Dr. Deber has written extensively on a wide range of health-care issues and is a member of the Board of the Canadian Health Economics Research Association.

Michael Decter is Deputy Minister of Health for Ontario. He has wide experience in management consulting, primarily with a concern for health activities. Mr. Decter served as Chief Negotiator for the Government of Ontario in the 1990-91 negotiations with the Ontario Medical Association.

W. John S. Marshall is Chief of Staff at Kingston General Hospital. He is Chairman of the Ontario Medical Association's Committee on Economics and was a member of the Ontario Ministry of Health's Task Force on the Use and Provision of Medical Services.

Raynald Pineault is Professor and Chairman of the Department of Social and Preventive Medicine at the Université de Montréal. He has researched and written on a wide range of health-related topics, and his current interests reflect a concern for the way in which hospitals, public health units and physicians conduct their activities, and how this may change or develop.

Duncan G. Sinclair is Vice-Principal (Health Sciences) and Dean of the Faculty of Medicine at Queen's University. Dr. Sinclair has served as a member of the Ministry of Health's Steering Committee for Review of the Public Hospitals Act and was Chairman of the Task Force on Governance.

Joan P.H. Watson has been recognized for her experience as a consumer advocate, significantly with the CBC, as Chairperson of the Canadian Medical Association Task Force on the Allocation of Health Care Resources in Canada and as a member of the Premier's Council on Health Strategy for Ontario.

Christel A. Woodward is Professor in the Department of Clinical Epidemiology and Biostatistics, a member of the Department of Psychiatry as well as the Program for Educational Development and an Associate of the Centre for Health Economics and Policy Analysis in the Faculty of Health Sciences at McMaster University. Dr. Woodward researches and writes in the area of health and medical education. She continues to maintain contact with the Health Encounter Pilot Project.

Stephanie Woolhandler is Assistant Professor of Medicine at Harvard Medical School and Staff Physician in the Department of Medicine at the Cambridge Hospital. Dr. Woolhandler is the founder and National Coordinator of the Physicians for a National Health Program. Her interests lie in the area of financing health care.